Basics of Comprehensive IVUS-Guided PCI

Junko Honye
Editor

Basics of Comprehensive IVUS-Guided PCI

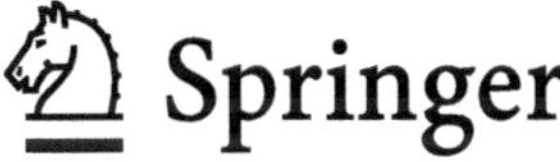

Editor
Junko Honye
Department of Cardiovascular Medicine
Kikuna Memorial Hospital
Yokohama, Kanagawa, Japan

ISBN 978-981-19-5660-7 ISBN 978-981-19-5658-4 (eBook)
https://doi.org/10.1007/978-981-19-5658-4

This English edition was published as a co-edition with its original Japanese language edition, PCI de tsukai taosu IVUS tettei katuyoujutu, copyright © 2020 by Medical View Co., Ltd., Tokyo Japan.

The translation was done with the help of artificial intelligence (machine translation by the service DeepL.com). A subsequent human revision was done primarily in terms of content.

This Springer imprint is published by the registered company Springer Nature Singapore Pte Ltd.
The registered company address is: 152 Beach Road, #21-01/04 Gateway East, Singapore 189721, Singapore

Preface to the First Edition

The Japanese are the happiest people in the world when it comes to intravascular imaging. Perhaps it was this sense of security that led to the question, "Isn't CAG a little disdainful?" It is also true that there is a sense of crisis.

It goes without saying that CAG is the most basic of all, and even in Japan, where intravascular imaging is so well developed, it is necessary to thoroughly review CAG before looking at IVUS. Stent size, length, and other PCI strategies should be determined to some extent based on CAG. In addition, distribution of plaque, plaque characteristics, and remodeling pattern of the lesion should be predicted in advance. After all procedures are completed, CAG and IVUS should be reviewed many times, including when PCI strategy is changed after IVUS observation, and operators can improve their reading skills of both CAG and IVUS by repeating the steady process of asking why CAG was not read correctly before PCI. Therefore, it is forbidden to say, "I will decide PCI strategies by looking at IVUS" in live demonstrations.

Why is IVUS necessary for PCI? It's about consideration, prediction, and verification, and that leads to high-quality PCI.

Consideration: Even if the severity of stenosis on CAG looks similar, those pathogenesis and plaque characteristics vary from case to case, and it is necessary to consider what can happen inside of the vessel by forcibly dilating the culprit lesion. We should develop PCI strategy that maximizes the effect by considering the mechanism of vessel dilation.

Prediction: Although complications may occur with some frequency as a result of PCI, their likelihood can be predicted from IVUS findings, and PCI strategies can be developed to reduce complications. If a complication unfortunately occurs, they can be anticipated in advance and dealt with calmly.

Verification: IVUS is an excellent learning tool, and it is important to verify "whether PCI procedures were adequately done or not" at the end of the PCI.

This book belongs to the category of "PCI" rather than "intravascular imaging," and is intended to help operators and cath lab staff with a basic knowledge of IVUS to maximize their ability to perform high-quality PCI. Therefore, specific techniques of PCI for complex lesions are also explained. IVUS is still a mainstream auxiliary diagnostic method for PCI because it provides a complete picture of the blood vessel. In the future, IVUS with higher frequency and resolution is expected to be marketed, and I strongly feel that IVUS still has a high potential.

I would like to express my gratitude to the doctors who wrote this book in spite of their busy schedules, and to Ms. Mayuko Yamada and everyone at Medical View for their efforts in publishing this book.

Yokohama, Japan Junko Honye
August 2015

Preface to the Second Edition

More than five years have passed since the first edition of *The Comprehensive Use of IVUS* was released in 2015. During the past 5 years, there have been significant advances in the IVUS itself: (1) introduction of higher frequencies, (2) introduction of high-speed pullback, and (3) introduction of IVUS catheters specifically designed for CTO.

1. High frequency

   With the availability of 60-MHz IVUS catheters from various companies, it has become common practice to use 60-MHz IVUS for PCI for open vessels. The improved resolution allows for clearer visualization of the inside of the plaque, including plaque rupture images, and also preserves deep penetration, emphasizing the advantages of IVUS.
2. High-speed pullback

   In addition to the conventional automatic pullback of 0.5 to 1 mm/s at 40 MHz, ACIST offers high-speed pullbacks of 2.5, 5, and 10 mm/s, and Terumo offers high-speed pullbacks of 3, 6, and 9 mm/s. This has advantages such as shortening the ischemic time, but on the other hand, it requires time and effort to stop operators' hands and review after the pullback is completed. In our hospital, we still use a pullback speed at 1 mm/s because we can select the landing zone and decide the size of the device while viewing the live pullback image, and then move it manually for marking technique.
3. IVUS catheter specialized for CTO

   In CTO, a catheter with a short distance between the IVUS transducer and the tip is preferred, but the IVUS catheter itself needs to be moved, which is a problem for operability. Recently, the AnteOwl WR ®, which has a short monorail tip and allows the transducer to be moved within the sheath, has been introduced. In this book, the technique using AnteOwl WR ® is described in detail, and we are pleased that the options for CTO cases have been expanded.

In this second edition, the updated data on IVUS and the specific use of high-frequency IVUS are explained more clearly than in the first edition. In addition, the number of articles related to "calcified lesions," "complications," and "CTO," which have been requested, has been greatly increased, and how to use IVUS to treat complex lesions more safely and effectively has been comprehensively explained. We are proud to say that this book is the result of combined efforts of IVUS experts in Japan, and our desire to provide patients by comprehensively reading both CAG and IVUS images and performing high-quality PCI has not changed. I would like to express my gratitude to all the doctors who took time out of their busy schedules to write this book, and to Ms. Mayuko Yamada and everyone at Medical View for their efforts in publishing this book.

Yokohama, Japan
October 2020

Junko Honye

Contents

Response of the Cath Lab Staff

Nobuyuki Soeda

Points for Comprehensive Use

- Understand the target case and then select an appropriate IVUS catheter.
- Understand the information the doctor is looking for, and anticipate.
- Understand complications.
- Understand the "trick" of IVUS and look at IVUS images.

IVUS-guided PCI is now commonly used in most cath labs. In this chapter, we discuss how medical staff can participate in the treatment as a member of the team.

1 Selection of an IVUS Catheter

IVUS systems currently available are made by Phillips, Boston Scientific, Terumo, Assist, and Nipro. There are two types of IVUS systems: mechanical scanning type (OptiCross™ 40 MHz/60 MHz: Boston Scientific, AltaView® 60MHz/AnteOwl WR™ 40 MHz: Terumo, Revolution® 45 MHz: Phillips, Kodama® 60 MHz: Assist and Dualpro™ 50 MHz: Nipro), and phased-array type (EagleEye 20 MHz/Visions® PV.018: Phillips). Only Phillips offers both types (Table 1).

Supplementary Information The online version contains supplementary material available at https://doi.org/10.1007/978-981-19-5658-4_1.

N. Soeda (✉)
Department of Clinical Engineering, Hoshi General Hospital, Koriyama, Fukushima, Japan
e-mail: n26soeda@nifty.com

J. Honye (ed.), *Basics of Comprehensive IVUS-Guided PCI*,
https://doi.org/10.1007/978-981-19-5658-4_1

Table 1 Types of IVUS and differences in specifications

	Phased-array type	Mechanical type				
	Phillips	Phillips	Boston	Terumo	ACIST	Nipro
Imaging system	s5™	s5™	Polaris™	VISICUBE®	HDi®	Makoto™
Imaging catheter	Eagle Eye® Visonos®PV.018	Revolution®	OptiCross™	AltaView® AnteOwl WR™	Kodama®	Dualpro™
Frequency	20 MHz	45 MHz	40–60 MHz	40–60 MHz	40–60 MHz	50 MHz
Flame rate	–	30	30	90	60	30
Pullback speed	0.5–1 mm/s	0.5–1 mm/s	0.5–8 mm/s	0.5–9 mm/s	0.5–10 mm/s	0.5–2 mm/s

2 Preparation

2.1 For Regular Use

There are different ways to use IVUS in different cases, and the cath lab staff needs to understand these characteristics and prepare them for each particular case. Each IVUS catheter has its special characteristics, which are suitable for regular use, in cases with large vessel diameter, and chronic total occlusion (CTO).

I think that Boston Scientific OptiCross™ and Terumo AltaView® 60MHz are the most suitable for regular use. The reason is that they can display two images on the same screen called "Dualview" with one pullback, measure distal reference and proximal reference segments, measure lesion length, and instantly provide lots of information that the operator wants (Fig. 1).

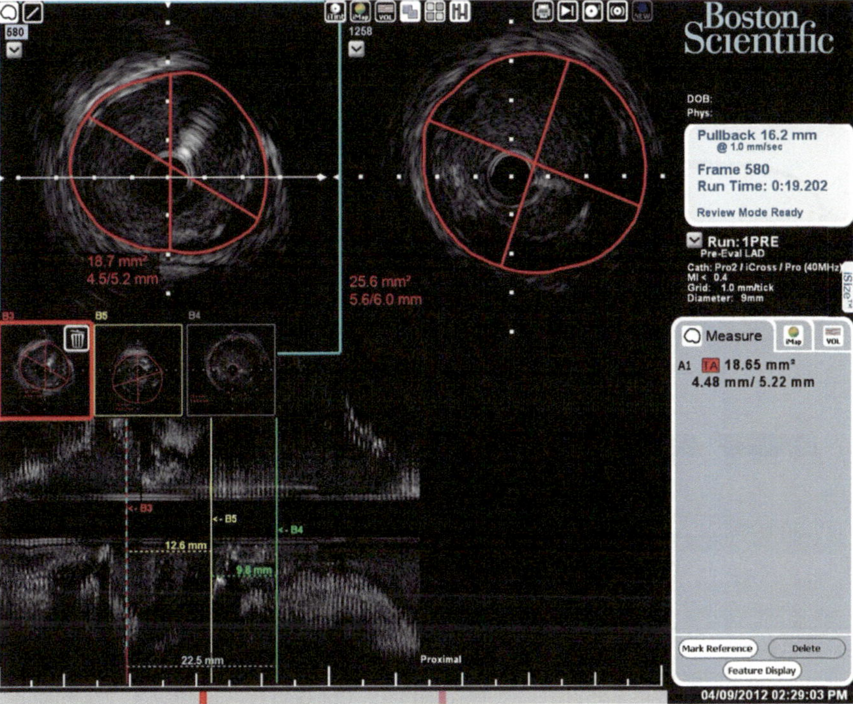

Fig. 1 Dualview of Boston Scientific OptiCross™

2.2 *For Cases with Large Vessel Diameters*

In patients with large vessel diameters, a low-frequency catheter should be selected. A catheter with higher frequency provides a shallower depth of penetration so that it is not able to demonstrate the whole vessel size and all information you need. Especially, 20 MHz Visions® PV .018 catheter (Philips) provides images with deep penetration and is effective even in large vessels such as iliac arteries (Fig. 2).

2.3 *For CTO Cases*

In cases with CTO, good crossability and a short distance from the tip to the transducer are absolute requirements. In particular, during IVUS-guided CTO, because a long-tip IVUS catheter may enlarge the false lumen, the total stent length would be very long even if the true lumen is captured. On the other hand, Terumo's AnteOwl WR™ has the shortest tip length (8 mm) among current IVUS catheters with long monorail, which is ideal for CTO cases (Fig. 3). In addition, since frame

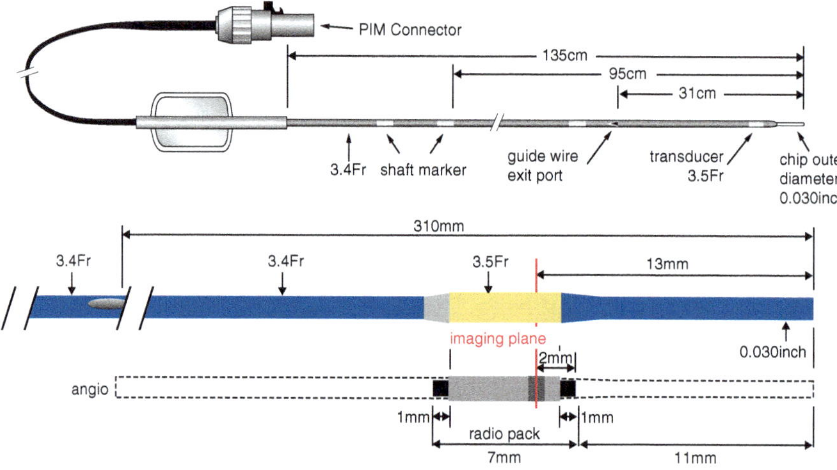

Catheter Size			Frequency (MHz)	Effective length (cm)	Minimum compatible guiding catheter (Fr)	Max. compatible guidewire (inch)	Maximum visible diameter (mm)
Chip outer diameter (inch)	Distal shaft (Fr)	Proximal shaft (Fr)					
0.03	3.4	3.4	20	135	6	0.018	24

Fig. 2 Visions® PV .018 : 20 MHz phased array IVUS imaging catheter

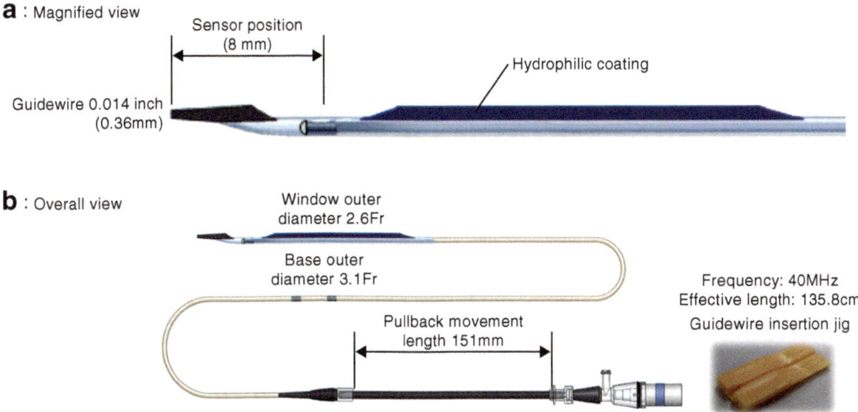

Fig. 3 AnteOwl WR™

rate and pullback speed differ depending on the IVUS system, it is necessary to select an adequate IVUS system, for example, with a higher frame rate and faster pullback speed in cases in which ischemic time needs to be shortened such as LMT lesions. However, if only pullback speed is faster without using a higher frame rate, it may lead to measurement errors so they should be cautious about them (Table 1).

2.4 Notes on the Overall Preparation (Video S1)

There are several pitfalls in preparation as well. The first is priming an IVUS catheter with mechanical type. Mechanical scan IVUS requires priming, and the first time flush with saline is crucial. When priming with high pressure, saline overtakes air, and microbubbles are created in the line. Once the microbubbles are created, it is difficult to remove them, and air causes ultrasound attenuation during image observation.

Here's the Trick

The trick is to perform priming as slowly as possible with lower pressure, as you fill an artificial heart-lung circuit. For this reason, it is important not to use a small syringe for priming and not to apply strong pressure. If you use a large syringe and fill it slowly at low pressure, microbubbles are very unlikely to be created in the tube (Fig. 4).

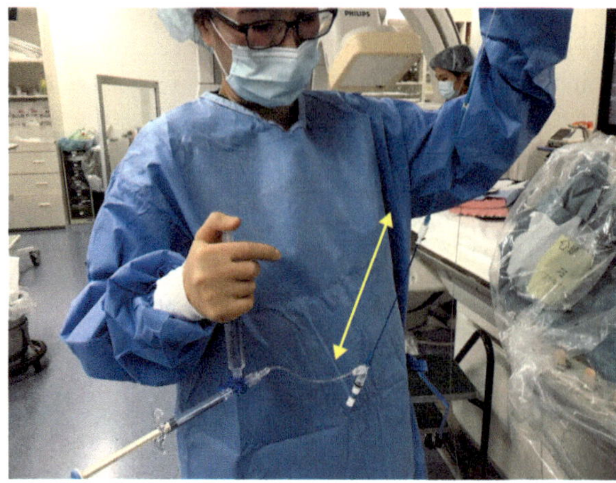

Fig. 4 Tips for priming. (**a**) Magnified view. (**b**) Overall view

3 During the Procedure

3.1 Environment Setting

The role of co-medical staff during a procedure is to set up the environment. IVUS observation before PCI may cause hemodynamic changes due to ischemia, the appearance of symptoms, and ECG changes. It is necessary to pay attention to all biological information such as hemodynamics, and it is essential to set up a safe environment.

3.2 Understand What Information the Doctor Wants

Next, it is important to understand what an operator wants to know. In general, as mentioned at the beginning of this chapter, baseline IVUS before PCI is used to:

1. Provide orientation during catheter insertion.
2. Record from a distal segment to the ostium as a control observation.
3. Marking at a distal reference segment, and bookmark.
4. Bookmark and marking at the culprit lesion.
5. Marking at a proximal reference segment, and bookmark.
6. Measure the length from a distal reference segment to the lesion, and the proximal reference segment (diameter and length) and determine the size of the STENT.
7. If one STENT cannot cover the whole lesion, measure the distance between the distal reference segment and the side branch, and the distance between the proximal reference segment to the side branch, and then determine stent size. The key to this process is how quickly it is performed.

3.2.1 Read IVUS Images to Prevent Complications

From there, it is still necessary to read IVUS images to prevent complications. For this purpose, it is important to understand the anatomical orientation of the coronary artery, such as whether the lesion is hard, what kind of IVUS findings are likely to cause perforation, and whether there is a possibility of cardiac tamponade when perforation occurs (Figs. 5, 6, and 7).

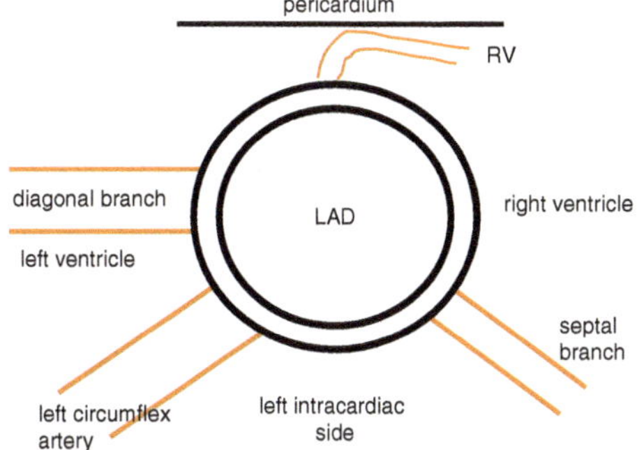

- IVUS depicts an image looking from the aortic side toward the apex
- Pericardium is essentially a cardiac surface side
- The LAD is 90° clockwise from the pericardium on the right ventricular side
- Ventricular side in the opposite direction from the pericardium
- Diagonal branch side at 90° counter-clockwise from the pericardium
- i.e., on the cardiac surface side in a 90° clockwise direction from a diagonal branch.
- Right ventricular side in the opposite direction.
- Left ventricular side at 90° direction counter-clockwise

Fig. 5 Orientation of the left anterior descending artery (LAD)

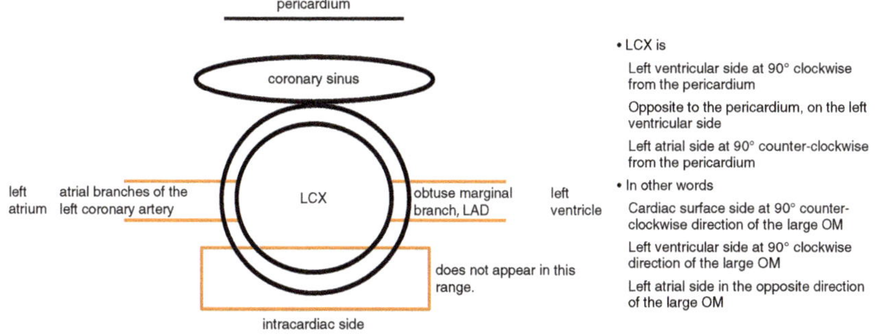

Fig. 6 Orientation of the left circumflex artery (LCX)

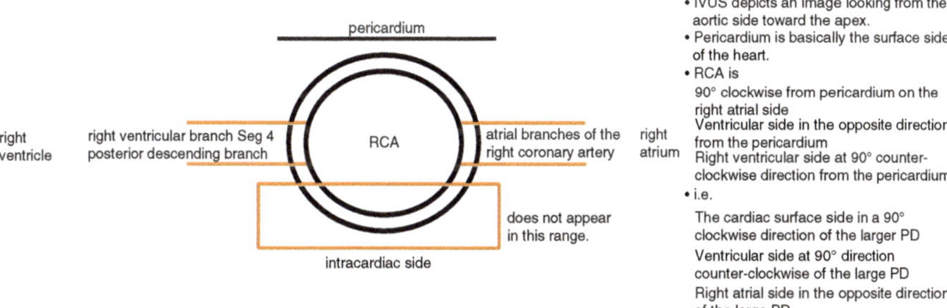

Fig. 7 Orientation of the right coronary artery (RCA)

3.2.2 Find Attenuated Plaque

It is important to recognize attenuated plaque and to provide information to the operator on whether the plaque contains lipid, and whether there is a possibility of slow flow or no-reflow after dilation when the attenuated plaque is long in the longitudinal view (Fig. 8). After STENT implantation, it is also very important to inform the operators whether the STENT is properly dilated, whether the STENT is nicely apposed to the vessel (Fig. 9), and how much lumen area is obtained, as these

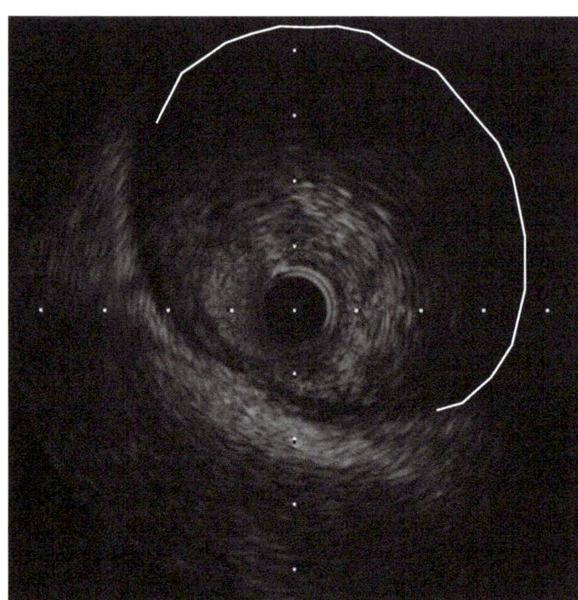

Fig. 8 Attenuated plaque

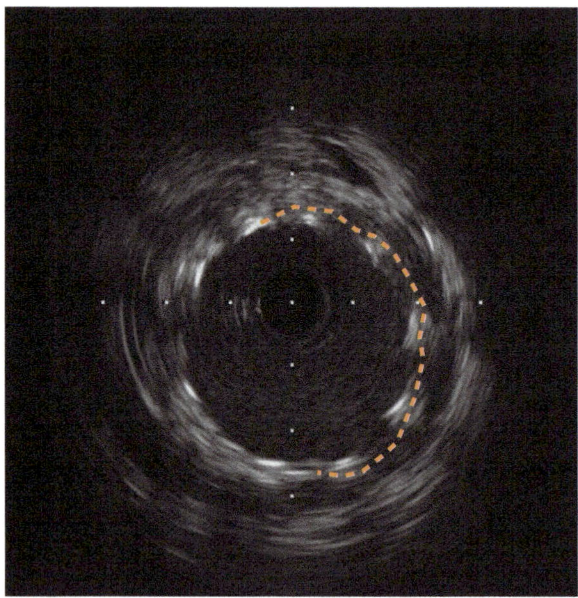

Fig. 9 Incomplete stent apposition

factors are related to the patient's long-term prognosis. In addition, it is necessary to set up an environment in which there is no measurement error due to coaxial (Fig. 10) and nonuniform rotational distortion (NURD, Fig. 11), which are unique deceptions to IVUS itself, and to inform the operators of probable measurement errors.

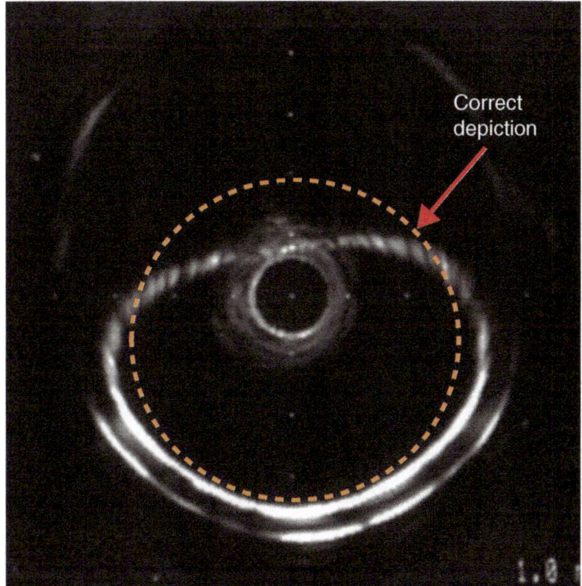

Fig. 10 Coaxial. Vessels are ovalized in flexion

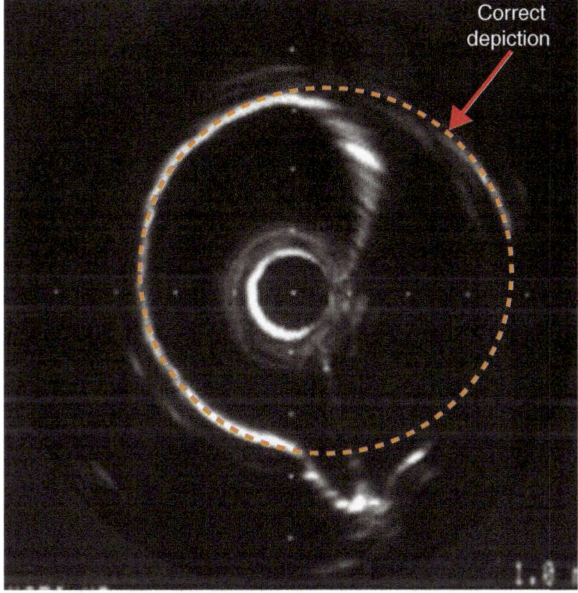

Fig. 11 NURD. Occurs only in mechanical type, image stretches in the lateral direction

4 After the PCI

The postoperative period is to analyze the data. I believe that the analysis of these data is the work of the co-medical staff. By having the co-medical staff analyze parts of the data that could not be analyzed during the procedure, you will be able to read imaging information more deeply, and his/her interest in IVUS will grow. Naturally, it is desirable for people who were involved in the procedure to take responsibility for data analysis. Particularly in cases where complications have occurred, it is important to communicate with operators, analyze imaging data thoroughly, investigate the cause of complications, and share that information with operators so that IVUS images should be reviewed until it is satisfactory, the same situations can be handled when it occurs. By continuing to do so, we believe that IVUS information will be created in another sense.

Advice
IVUS is a device that provides imaging information, not a therapeutic device. How to use IVUS in a safe environment is up to physicians and other co-medical staff, and complications due to the use of IVUS are out of the question. It is up to physicians and co-medical staff to understand the characteristics of catheters and therapeutic devices and to work hard to select an appropriate catheter and device for each case. The most important point is to share information on whether the patient can be safely treated with IVUS before PCI, such as the target lesion, severity of the disease, and whether the hemodynamic status is stable. To achieve this, all the staff in the cath lab needs to understand and share patient information in preoperative conferences.

How to Apply Artifacts during PCI?

Shinjo Sonoda

Points for Comprehensive Use

- To interpret IVUS accurately, it is important to extract a clean image with fewer artifacts.
- In recent years, high-resolution IVUS has been developed, resulting in clear images with less noise, but adequate saline flushing in advance is essential and should not be neglected.
- Some artifacts can be avoided and some cannot, but the characteristics and causes of each must be accurately understood, and when avoidable, careful consideration must be given to devise settings and catheter manipulation.
- Understanding how artifact occurs is also important in performing secure PCI.

1 What Is an Artifact?

These are images that are not intended or do not exist (false images). Artifacts that should be differentiated can be divided into the five major categories shown in Table 1.

Supplementary Information The online version contains supplementary material available at https://doi.org/10.1007/978-981-19-5658-4_2.

S. Sonoda (✉)
Department of Cardiovascular Medicine, Faculty of Medicine, Saga University, Saga, Japan
e-mail: ssonoda@cc.saga-u.ac.jp

J. Honye (ed.), *Basics of Comprehensive IVUS-Guided PCI*,
https://doi.org/10.1007/978-981-19-5658-4_2

Table 1 Artifacts to be differentiated

Not avoidable	1. Due to the physical properties of ultrasound (echo) (Fig. 1)
	• Ring down • Blood speckle • Side lobe • Acoustic shadow • Reverberation • Attenuation
	2. Due to the effect on the heartbeat (Fig. 2)
	• Motion artifacts in the short- and long-axes directions
	3. Caused by the apparatus
	• Guidewire artifact • Guiding catheter artifact
Avoidable	4. Caused by the operation (Fig. 3)
	• Uneven rotation (NURD) • Air bubbles
	5. Other (Fig. 4)
	• Position artifact • Accordion

1.1 Glossary of Artifact Terms

Ring Down
Acoustic noise is produced in the proximity of a transducer, resulting from large amplitude vibrations of the piezoelectric element. Also called "proximal distance sound field crack" (turbulence). Stronger with electronic scanning than with mechanical scanning.

Side Lobe
Echogenic, linear, or curvilinear artifacts appear from echo images of structures with strong acoustic impedance.

Blood Speckle
Echo noise scattered from red blood cells obscures the luminal boundaries.

Acoustic Shadow
Calcification and strong echo-reflective objects such as guidewires, stents, and other artificial structures cause posterior shade defects.

Reverberation
In structures with a strong acoustic impedance (calcification, stents, etc.), double and triple echoes are often seen with equal spacing.

Attenuation
Even in the absence of a strong reflection, the echoes in the plaque may be attenuated due to absorption and scattering of ultrasound, and the backward view may not be observed. It is often seen in lesions of acute coronary syndromes, which are unstable plaques and may cause slow flow/no reflow during PCI.

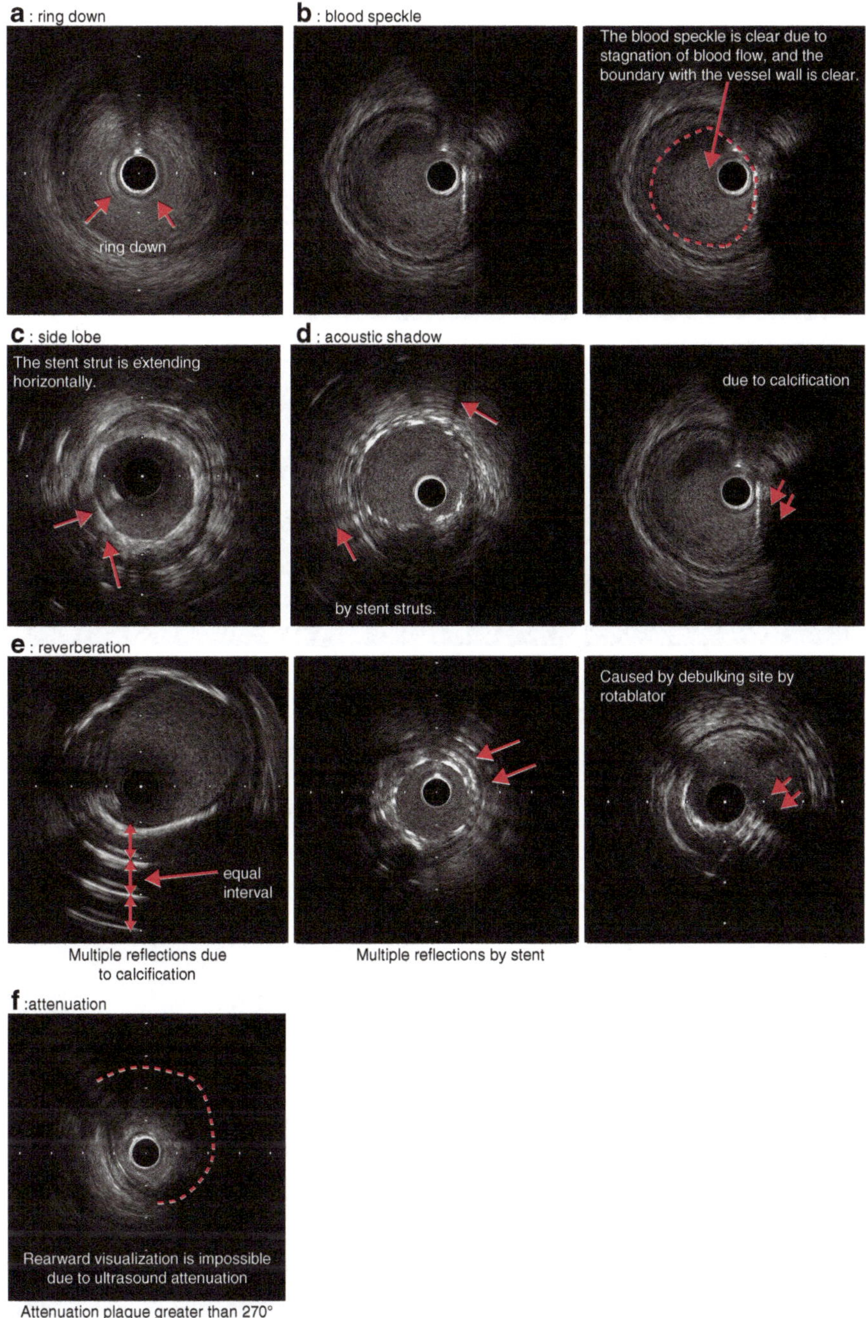

Fig. 1 Due to the physical properties of ultrasound. (**a**) Ring down. (**b**) Blood speckle. (**c**) Side lobe. (**d**) Acoustic shadow. (**e**) Reverberation. (**f**) Attenuation

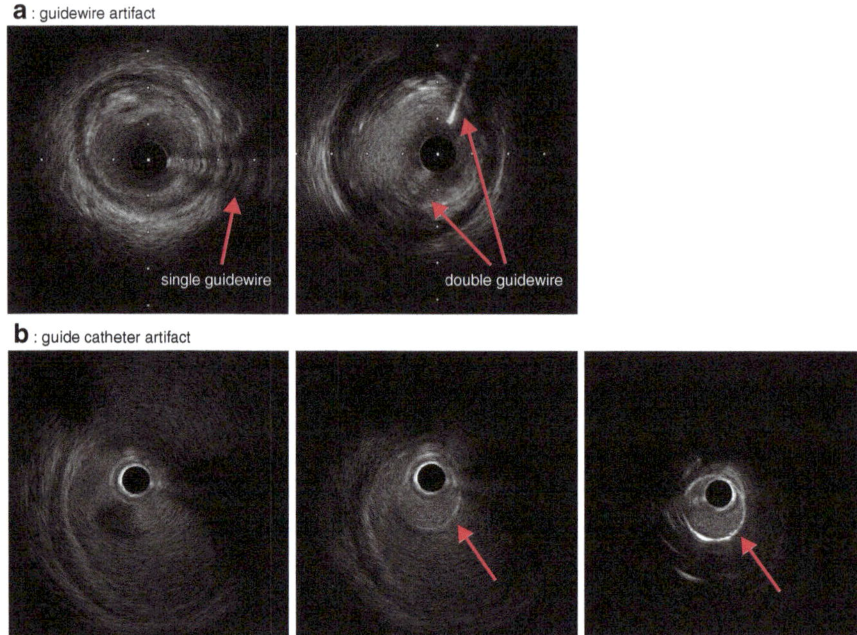

Fig. 2 Attributed to devices. (**a**) Guidewire artifact. (**b**) Guide catheter artifact

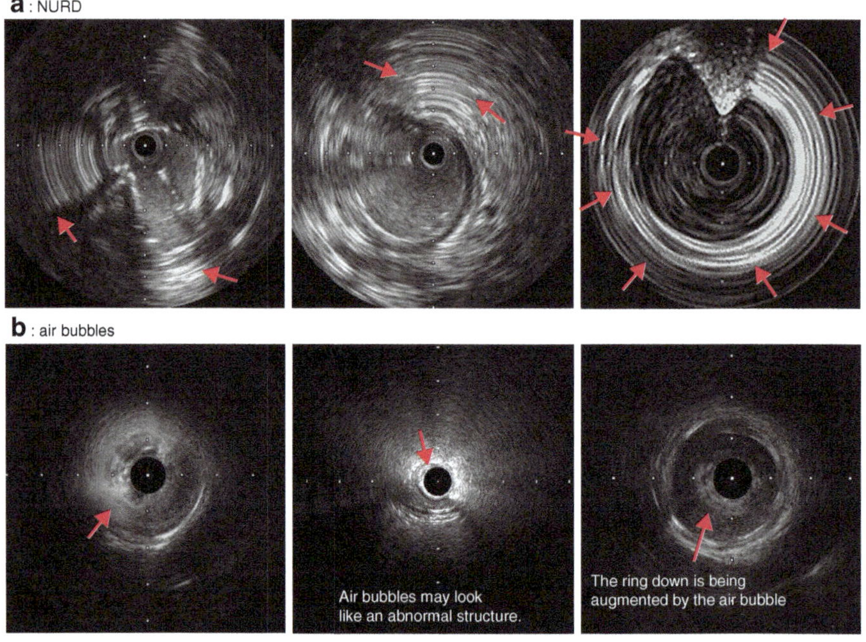

Fig. 3 Operation induced. (**a**) NURD (Movie: Video S1). (**b**) Air bubbles (Movie: Video S2)

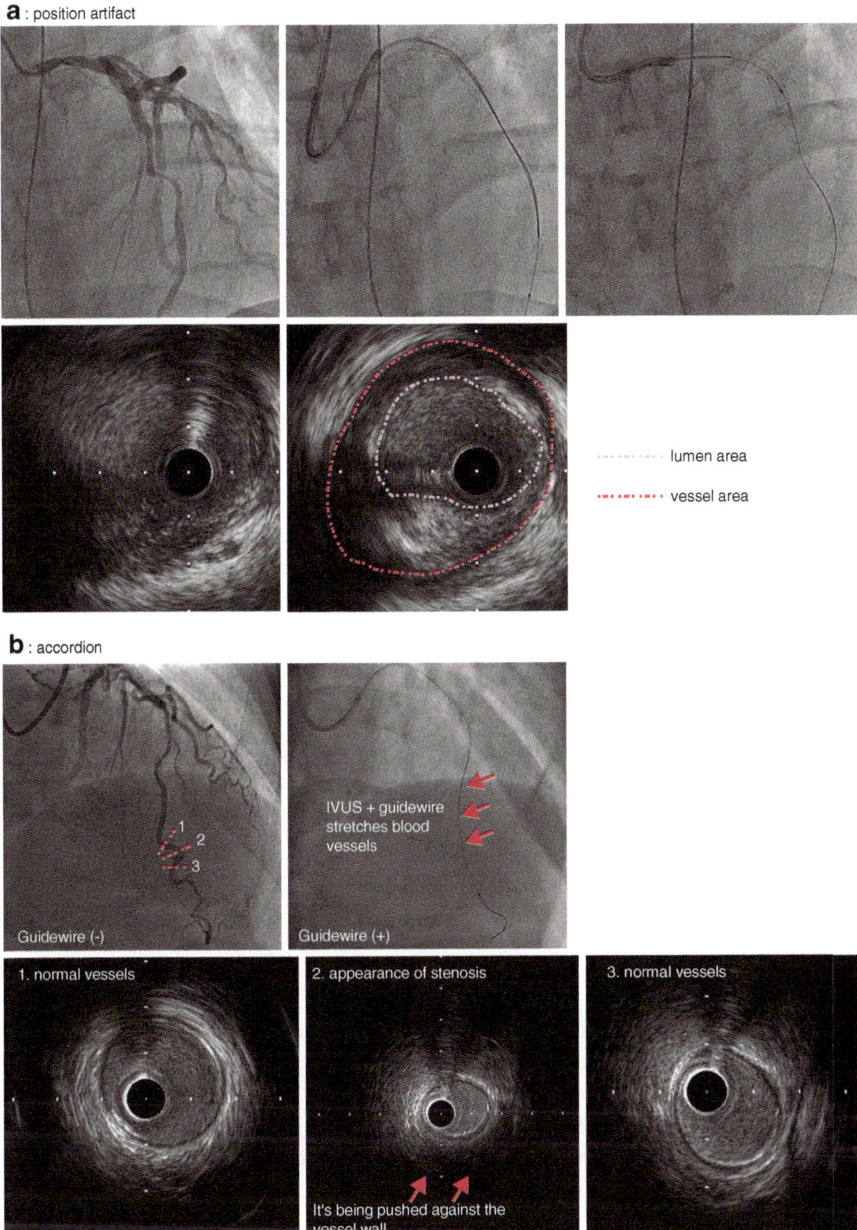

Fig. 4 Others. (**a**) Position artifact. 1. Angiographic findings of the left coronary artery. 2. Uneven positioning of the IVUS catheter due to the guiding catheter and oblique slice cross-section at the ostium. 3. Coaxiality between guiding catheter and IVUS was maintained and correct cross-sectional images were obtained. Pink dotted line: Lumen area. Red dotted line: Vessel area. (**b**) Accordion (Movie: Video S3). It is often seen in vessels with strong tortuosity. (**c**) Electrical noise. (**d**) Disconnection

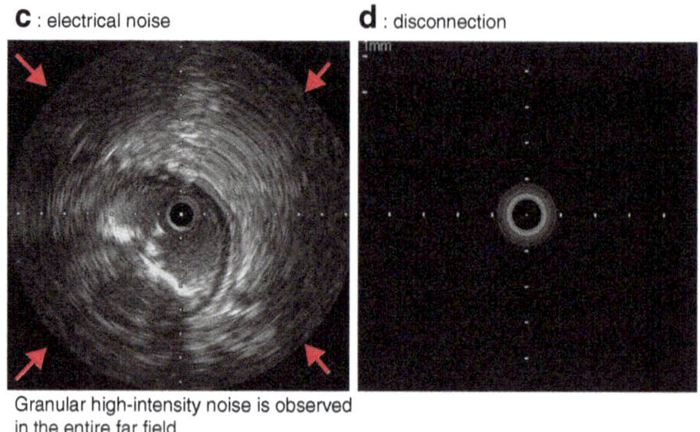

Fig. 4 (continued)

Motion Artifacts

This is an artifact that appears due to the effect of cardiac beat, and blurring of the image is observed in both the short and long axes of the vessel. In some cases, it is possible to adjust the coaxial and the position of the guiding catheter.

Guidewire Artifact

The guidewire, a strong echo-reflective object, causes an acoustic shadow behind it, which affects the quantitative and qualitative observation of the lumen and vessel.

Guiding Catheter Artifact

In the entrance of the right and left coronary arteries, deep insertion of the guiding catheter may cause a concentric, high-echo intensity structure at the ostium, resulting in inadequate observation of the lumen area and possibly missing stenosis or injury at the entrance. At the end of the procedure, the guiding catheter should be removed from the ostium and observed again. Recently, it has become possible to obtain information on the entry site using some specific guide extension catheters.

Non-Uniform Rotational Distortion (NURD)

For mechanical scanning IVUS catheters, uneven rotation of the transducer is the cause. The most common causes are strong tortuosity of the coronary artery, bending of the IVUS catheter inside and outside the body, the angle between the guiding catheter entrance and the vessel wall, and excessive closure of the Y-connector. With the evolution of IVUS catheters, strong NURD is less common. However, NURD is still seen in complex lesions with severe calcium and tortuosity.

Air Bubbles

It is frequently observed when the saline flush is inadequate. As a precaution, careful flushing should be done externally. If the IVUS catheter is not removed and flushed inside the body, air embolism may occur, resulting in chest pain and prolonged ST-segment elevation on ECG.

Position Artifacts

In ostial lesions such as the left main trunk (LMT), the guiding catheter is often not inserted coaxially with the vessel from the beginning. In that case, the vessel will be elliptical due to the oblique cross-section, which overestimates the vessel and lumen areas. The measurement of the lumen area is an important point in the evaluation of the indication for PCI in LMT.

Accordion

When a guidewire is inserted into a bent coronary artery, the vessel is stretched and folded, giving the appearance of plaque or stenosis. It is useful to be familiar with the characteristics of the image. It is important to confirm that the stenosis is false stenosis caused by the accordion phenomenon by performing another angiography after the guidewire is finally removed.

Electrical Noise

Other medical electric devices in the room may cause electrical noise in the IVUS image (white powdery snow, radial lines). If the source of the noise can be identified, it can be avoided by switching off or moving the devices.

Catheter Disconnection

If the screen suddenly blacked out and only concentric catheter image are seen, there is a possibility of disconnection. In the case of complete disconnection, it is necessary to replace the catheter with a new IVUS catheter. First of all, keep in mind to check for a bad connection between the catheter and the transducer.

2 Know the NURD of High-Resolution (60 MHz) IVUS

As mentioned earlier, in the era of high-resolution IVUS, the appearance of NURD has become less common. The areas where NURD is observed are often highly bent and calcified, and NURD can cause errors in the measurement of vessel diameter and lumen diameter, leading to misjudgment of balloon size and endpoint. Therefore, caution is required.

3 Utilizing Hemocyte Echocardiography for PCI

A blood speckle is an artifact that is always present in the lumen of the vessels. Flushing with saline, half-diluted contrast medium, or low molecular weight dextran replaces the red blood cells with anechoic material and clarifies the boundary (negative contrast technique).

Blood speckles may be present between the stent and the lumen (stent under expansion) or within the media or extravascularly (dissection/hematoma), which is helpful in the diagnosis. The presence of incomplete stent apposition, dissection, or hematoma may lead to acute coronary occlusion and additional treatment may be necessary. In bifurcation lesions, the presence or absence of blood speckles within the lumen in the side branches can also be useful to determine side branch occlusions.

Because the blood speckle is useful in determining the boundary between the lumen and the vessel wall, it is very convenient to use the Dynamic Review function (available on several IVUS equipment), which allows repetitive review of several frames before and after.

4 Utilizing Guidewire Artifacts for PCI

A guidewire is an artifact that is always present in the vessel during PCI procedures. However, it creates an acoustic shadow on the back, which usually interfere with what we want to observe. On the other hand, the guidewire itself may be useful as a marker (of the side branch), and the run and position of the wire (guidewire bias) within the lumen are often useful as reference findings for treatment.

Advice
Artifacts are inherent in IVUS reading. It is important to understand and deal with their characteristics. Minimize artifacts, read IVUS based on the artifacts, and use them for PCI.

Suggested Readings

Mintz GS, Nissen SE, Anderson WD, et al. American college of cardiology clinical expert consensus document on standards for acquisition, measurement and reporting of intravascular ultrasound studies (IVUS). A report of the American College of cardiology task force on clinical expert consensus documents. J Am Coll Cardiol. 2001;37:1478–92.

Sonoda S. Artifacts. In: Kobayashi Y, Sonoda S, Morino Y, et al, editors. IVUS reading technique for PCI. Tokyo: Igaku Shoin; 2005. p. 22–7.

Notes on IVUS Catheter Manipulation

Junko Honye

Points for Comprehensive Use

- Use high-frequency IVUS for open-vessel PCI.
- Bleed air as slowly as possible during setup.
- When removing the IVUS catheter, pull it out slowly under fluoroscopic guidance.

An IVUS catheter is a precision machine that requires more than 1000 steps to complete. Although IVUS is covered by insurance in Japan, it is expensive as everybody knows. Therefore, it is necessary to feedback all the information obtained from IVUS to PCI procedures, including the crossability of the IVUS catheter itself. In addition, it is necessary to manipulate IVUS catheters correctly to obtain the highest-quality images as much as possible you can.

1 High-Frequency IVUS Used for PCI

In routine PCI, a 40–60 MHz high-frequency IVUS system is used. It is recommended to develop habits of interpreting IVUS images including not only vessel diameters but also blood cell speckles and extravascular structures.

J. Honye (✉)
Kikuna Memorial Hospital, Yokohama, Kanagawa, Japan
e-mail: jhonye@kmh.or.jp

J. Honye (ed.), *Basics of Comprehensive IVUS-Guided PCI*,
https://doi.org/10.1007/978-981-19-5658-4_3

2 Points for Catheter Setup

To obtain better images, fine air bubbles around the transducer should be removed. In the commonly used mechanical IVUS catheter, the setup is as follows:

1. Once the complete IVUS catheter is removed from the package, pull the imaging core out to the front.
2. Attach a 2.5-cc syringe in a straight line and flush as slowly as possible (over 10 s).
3. After the flush is completed, care should be taken to prevent air from entering the circuit, and the three-way stopcock used with the syringe for the flush should be turned off in the catheter's direction.
4. After the flush, the setup is complete when the pullback device is attached to the IVUS catheter and advance an imaging core to the tip of the catheter. After the setup is completed, one should not pull back the imaging core from the tip, because air will enter from the tip.
5. Flushing with the catheter in the coronary artery can induce air embolization, and care should be taken.

Advice
The authors have made a video and uploaded it to YouTube for your reference. YouTube (https://www.youtube.com/) → Search for "IVUS catheter preparation".

3 Precautions to be Taken When Advancing the Catheter

When advancing the IVUS catheter into a coronary artery, the catheter should be advanced to at least 10 mm distal to the lesion if possible, while confirming the tip of the catheter under fluoroscopic guidance. At this time, the authors advance the IVUS catheter into the coronary artery by rotating an imaging core, because the catheter itself has "stiffness" when the imaging core is rotated. However, if it is difficult to cross the lesion, forced advance of the IVUS catheter while rotating it may cause a catheter break.

The IVUS catheter should be kept straight from the guiding catheter to the pullback device without deflection (Fig. 1). Overtightening of a Y-connector or deflection of the catheter can cause NURD (nonuniform rotational distortion).

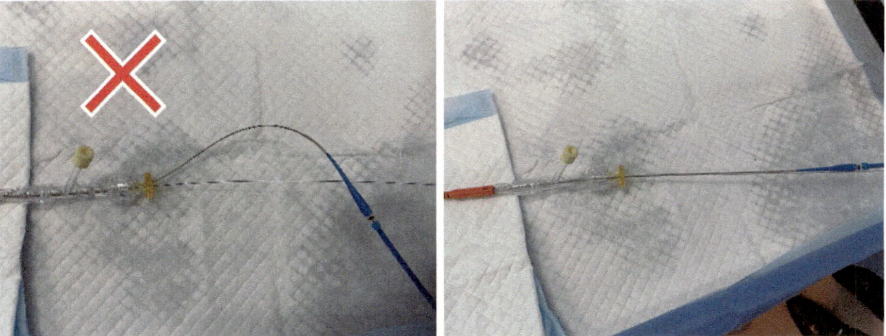

Fig. 1 The IVUS catheter should be kept straight from the guiding catheter

4 When the IVUS Catheter Does Not Cross the Lesion Before PCI

4.1 Cause

1. Severe calcification at the lesion or tight stenosis due to fibrous plaque.
2. Highly angulated lesion.

4.2 How to Deal with (Problem, etc.)

1. If the IVUS catheter does not pass, make a stronger backup force and try again to advance the catheter. It is not recommended to advance with vibrating the catheter, because it may damage the tip of the catheter. Then remove it and make lesion preparation with a Rotablator or a balloon.
2. This corresponds to a wide bifurcation angle of the circumflex artery from the left main trunk (Fig. 2a) angulated proximal right coronary artery. In a sheath-type catheter, the protective sheath tries to follow the vessel, whereas the rigid imaging core in the sheath tries to go straight. The tip of the imaging core is located near the exit port of the guidewire, which is structurally the most vulnerable part of the IVUS catheter and susceptible to bending. To avoid this, pull the imaging core back 2–3 cm (Fig. 2b), advance the entire catheter and then advance the imaging core again after the tip crosses the lesion (Fig. 2c).

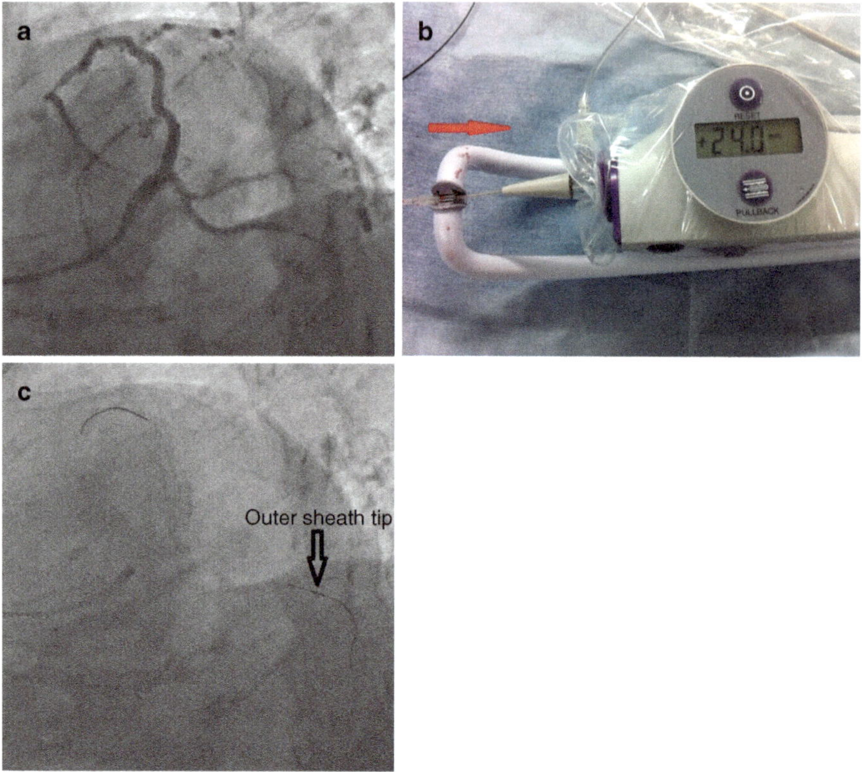

Fig. 2 Measures to be taken when the angle of the circumflex artery is very tight in this case. (**a**) The left circumflex with strong bifurcation angle. (**b**) Pull out the imaging core 2–3 cm from the tip. (**c**) Advance the IVUS catheter into the distal segment of the lesion, then advance the imaging core to the tip

5 When the IVUS Catheter Does Not Cross the Lesion After PCI

5.1 Cause

1. Stent under expansion: The tip of the IVUS catheter is caught with stent struts, especially at the bend.
2. If the proximal end of the stent is placed at angulated segments: The IVUS catheter tip is trapped in the stent edge at the outer curvature of the angulation, making it difficult to pass.
3. A flap of calcification: when dissection occurs in plaque with calcification, sometimes after Rotablator, and it blocks a lumen to pass.

5.2 *How to Deal with (Problem, etc.)*

1. After PCI, forced advancement of the IVUS catheter may cause damaged stent struts and should be avoided.
2. The IVUS catheter may be passed by altering the trajectory of its passage. Attempt to advance the IVUS catheter while pulling the guidewire slightly forward, or advance the guidewire and IVUS catheter together, or ask the patient to take a deep breath.
3. Perform post-dilatation with a balloon again, then the passage of the IVUS catheter should be attempted.
4. If the IVUS catheter still does not pass, the procedure should be terminated without final IVUS pullback.

6 Precautions During IVUS Image Recording

Chest pain and ST-T changes may occur during pullback, so an assistant or medical staff should pay attention to ECG and pressure monitoring. Fluoroscopic recording should always be performed when you start recording, so that the site of the pullback starting point should be clearly documented.

When using a Y-connector, it is advisable to hold the IVUS catheter itself with your fingertips as it may come loose during pullback.

First, perform an automatic pullback from the distal portion to the ostium, and then manually observe the lesion again as needed. Negative contrast with bolus injection of flush fluid through the guiding catheter, similar in principle to OCT, allows for a more detailed observation of the lesion (Fig. 3).

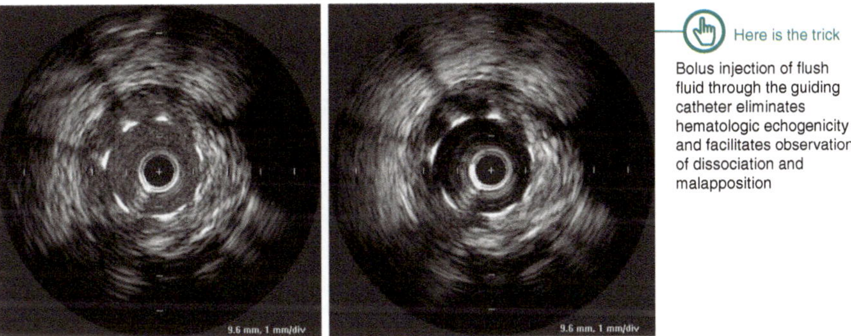

Fig. 3 Negative contrast method. Bolus injection of flush fluid through the guiding catheter eliminates hematologic echogenicity and facilitates observation of dissociation and malapposition

After the observation is completed and the IVUS catheter is withdrawn, the shaft of the IVUS catheter should be wiped with gauze and wetted with saline and the IVUS catheter should be flushed each time.

Points to Note When Removing the IVUS Catheter

At the end of the pullback, the imaging core is pulled out toward the front. If it is pulled out as it is, the exit port of the guidewire may get caught in the stent strut or the guidewire may become entangled at the tip of the guiding catheter because the distal part of the IVUS catheter is not stiff. Therefore, after completion of the pullback, the imaging core should be returned to the catheter tip, rotated, and removed under fluoroscopic guidance. Rotating the imaging core prevents the catheter tip from getting caught on the stent edge. If the speed of withdrawal is too fast, it may cause such problems. If the guidewire is deflected, pull the guidewire forward and pull the IVUS catheter alternately.

Comparison Between CAG and IVUS Findings

Tomohiko Teramoto

Points for Comprehensive Use

- IVUS may provide information that cannot be obtained with coronary angiography (CAG) alone.
- IVUS can play complementary roles when CAG findings alone are difficult to understand and determine.
- It is important to use imaging modalities in situations where it is difficult to understand the situations using CAG alone.

There is no disagreement that angiographic findings are the primary source of information in the decision-making process when performing PCI. However, to make PCI safer and more effective, CAG alone is insufficient, and IVUS is an essential device. Even in Europe, the USA, and other countries where the use of IVUS has lagged behind that of Japan in terms of cost in actual clinical practice, its usefulness has been gradually gaining ground in recent years. In this section, we compare characteristic findings observed by CAG with those observed by IVUS during PCI procedures.

1 Vascular Dissection

When the lumen of the vessel is enlarged by percutaneous old balloon angioplasty (POBA), a fissure is created in the plaque, and this fissure reaches the tunica media of the vessel, which is generally referred to as a dissection. If the fissure remains

T. Teramoto (✉)
Cardiovascular and General Medicine Center, Sakura General Hospital, Niwa County, Aichi, Japan
e-mail: tomo.tera@gmail.com

J. Honye (ed.), *Basics of Comprehensive IVUS-Guided PCI*,
https://doi.org/10.1007/978-981-19-5658-4_4

within the intima, it is called a tear. On CAG, it is often depicted as a slit-shaped shadow defect (Fig. 1), and on IVUS, it is observed that a crack enters the plaque from the vessel lumen, continuity of the vessel lumen is lost, and this crack reaches the intima, tunica media, and rarely adventitia (Fig. 2).

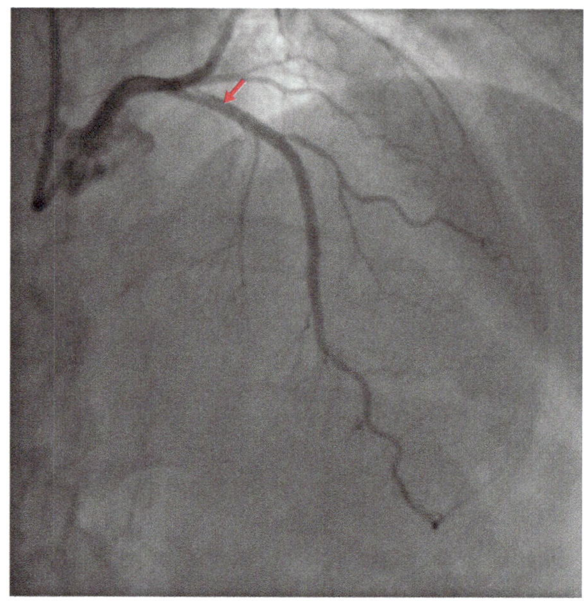

Fig. 1 Medial dissection formed by balloon angioplasty during PCI (red arrow). After additional balloon inflation of the proximal end of a stent placed in the distal left anterior descending artery (LAD), this dissection extended into the proximal LAD

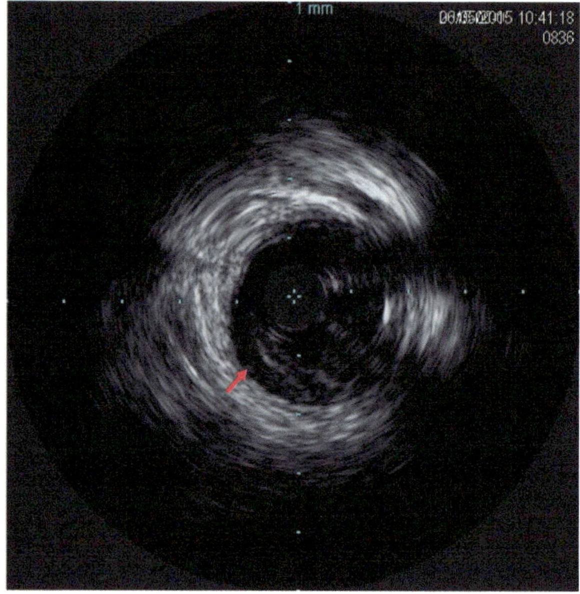

Fig. 2 IVUS image of the same region as the medial dissection observed in CAG. The crack extends from the lumen of the vessel into the plaque and media (red arrow). In this case, an additional stent was placed to cover the medial dissection

2 Thrombus

On CAG, a thrombus is represented by a translucent image (Fig. 3) and/or a vessel occlusion with a crab claw appearance. Often, floating thrombus can be also observed. When a floating thrombus appears as a contrast oozing over a long area (typically more than 5 mm), a large amount of thrombus is often present. In a case with acute myocardial infarction with an occluded culprit lesion that is suspicious of the presence of thrombus, thrombus may not be as troublesome to treat as it would be in a case where contrast is delayed but still visible into the periphery following guidewire passage. In general, the older the thrombus (organizing thrombus), the higher the echogenicity. Sometimes, mural thrombi can be difficult to differentiate from surrounding tissue (Fig. 4).

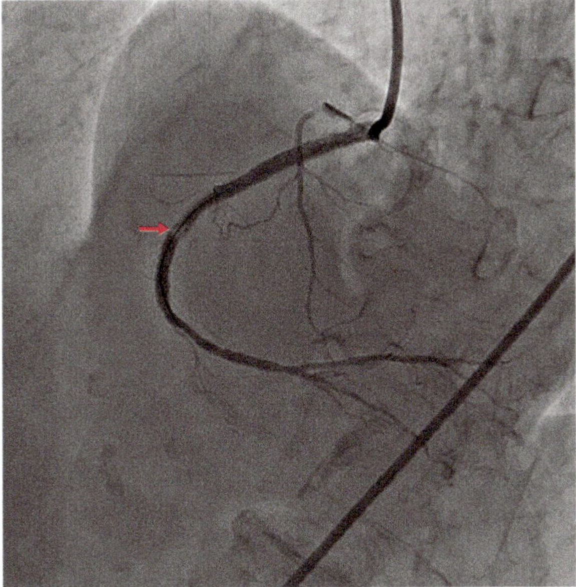

Fig. 3 Thrombus generated in the implanted stent during PCI. Although it may be difficult to recognize because of the guidewire, a fluoroscopic image can be seen inside the stent

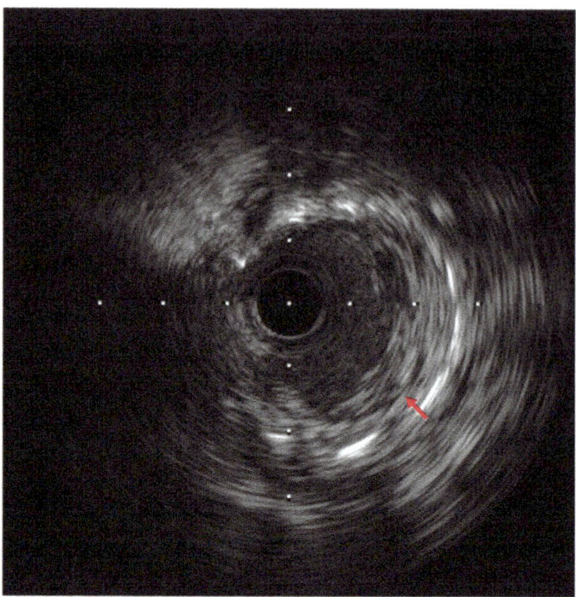

Fig. 4 IVUS of the same area as in Fig. 3 showing a thrombus with less echogenicity in the stent (red arrow). In this case, HIT (heparin-induced thrombocytopenia) was suspected, and thrombus aspiration, intracoronary infusion of urokinase, and argatroban were used to eliminate thrombus

3 Hematoma

Hematoma is the accumulation of blood in the dissected plane of tunica media after the formation of a vascular dissection. If luminal compression by the hematoma is mild, it may not be reflected as stenosis on CAG. On IVUS, a slightly hyperintense crescent-shaped area can be observed in the tunica media, reflecting the blood accumulation (Figs. 5 and 6). Pathologically, there are entries and re-entries between lumen and tunica media, but these are often not visible on IVUS.

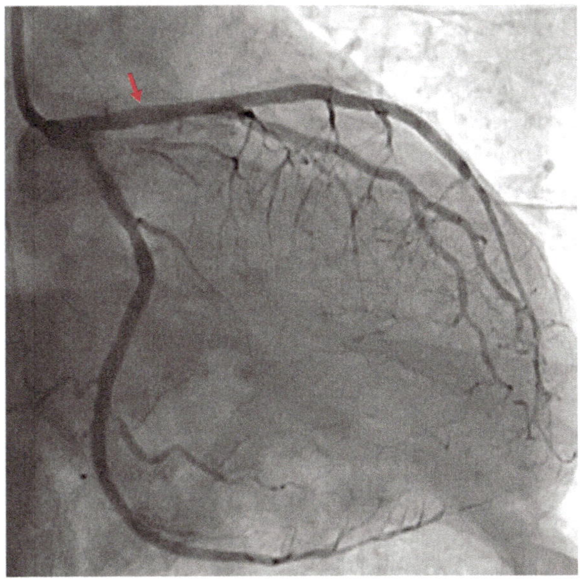

Fig. 5 CAG findings corresponding to the site of hematoma on IVUS (red arrow). No obvious abnormal findings can be detected by CAG

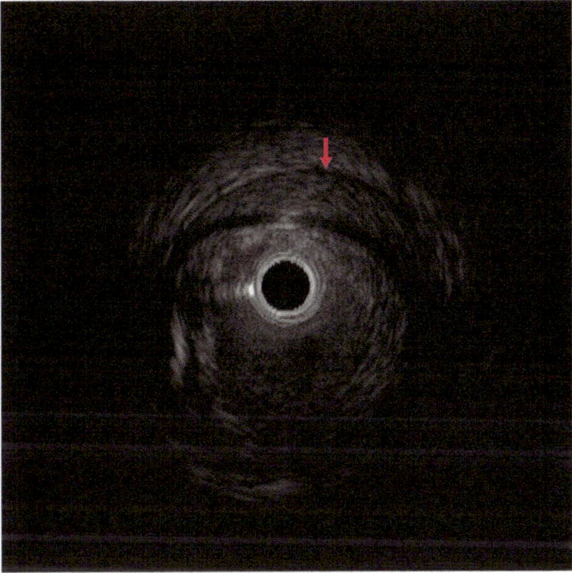

Fig. 6 IVUS image of the same site as Fig. 5. A hematoma was observed from the proximal end of the stent implanted in the distal to the proximal LAD (red arrow). Operators waited for about 20 minutes in the catheter room, and after confirming that there was no worsening of hematoma on repeat CAG, the patient was placed on follow-up observation

4 Calcification

As atherosclerosis progresses, calcium deposits are generally found in plaques to varying degrees. In heavily calcified lesions where the outline of the vessel can be recognized by calcium deposited on the adventitial side on CAG (Fig. 7), calcium itself is deeply deposited (deep calcium), and it is generally impossible to ablate with rotational atherectomy. In heavily calcified lesions with a superficial 360-degree circumferential calcification, the IVUS signal is most strongly enhanced and is seen as a layered reverberation posteriorly (Fig. 8).

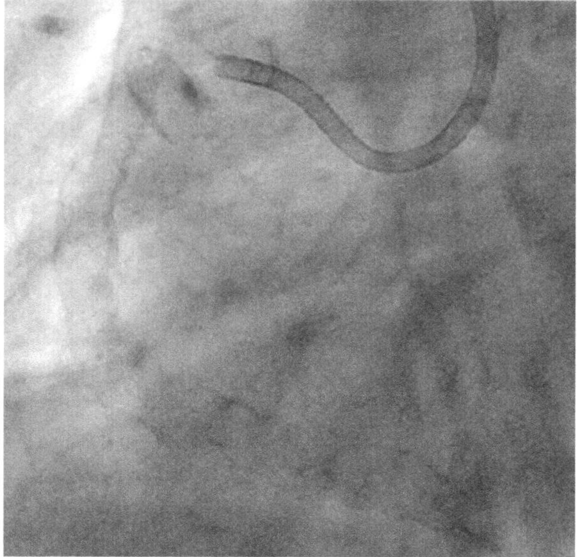

Fig. 7 Heavily calcified right coronary artery. The calcification itself was so severe that the outline of the vessel was recognized under fluoroscopy without the use of contrast media. In this case, there was no significant stenosis in the coronary artery, contrary to the high degree of calcification

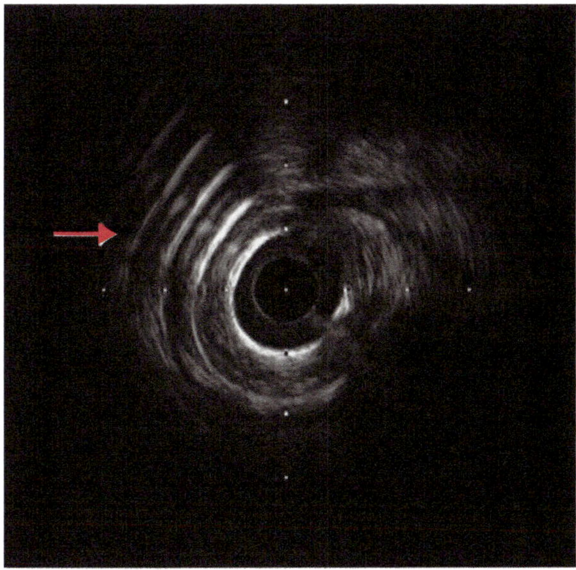

Fig. 8 Superficial calcification over approximately 270°. The lumen is about 2.0 × 2.0 mm. Multiple posterior echogenic signals are seen due to severe calcification (red arrow, reverberation phenomenon). In this case, after ablation with rotational atherectomy, stenting was performed and good dilation was successfully achieved

5 Plaque Deviation at the Stent Site

Because stenting itself does not reduce plaque volume, stenting of a soft, large amount of plaque often results in plaque compression and plaque prolapse through the stent struts into the lumen. This is referred to as plaque prolapse or plaque protrusion. CAG shows a light-filling defect and sometimes stenotic due to plaque prolapse in the stent. On IVUS, plaque prolapse in the stent can be seen as a slightly high echo signal. However, it is safer to use a distal protection device because high-pressure dilation may cause debris to be migrated into the distal bed, leading to a slow/no-reflow phenomenon. On the other hand, serious complications due to plaque prolapse are less common.

6 Incomplete Stent Apposition (Malapposition)

Incomplete stent apposition occurs when the stent implanted in the stenosis is not sufficiently apposed to the vessel wall. CAG often does not provide a clear picture, and IVUS can show stent struts floating in the lumen without being apposed on the intima (Fig. 9). Although malapposition of the distal part of the stent is not clinically problematic, malapposition of the proximal part may cause stent thrombosis, and it is preferable to dilate the proximal part of the stent as much as possible unless there is a strong risk for medial dissection due to additional dilatation.

Several typical findings that can occur during the course of PCI are compared between CAG and IVUS. Although these are a few of the phenomena that can occur during PCI procedure, they can lead to serious complications such as acute coronary occlusion if overlooked, and a thorough understanding of all of these phenomena is necessary to obtain maximum clinical benefit from PCI.

Advice

It is indisputable that the therapeutic strategy for PCI is based on CAG findings, but CAG is only a "shadow picture" and does not provide a complete picture of pathology occurring inside the vessel.

When it is difficult to understand what is happening based on CAG findings alone, it is important to be willing to observe using intravascular imaging modalities.

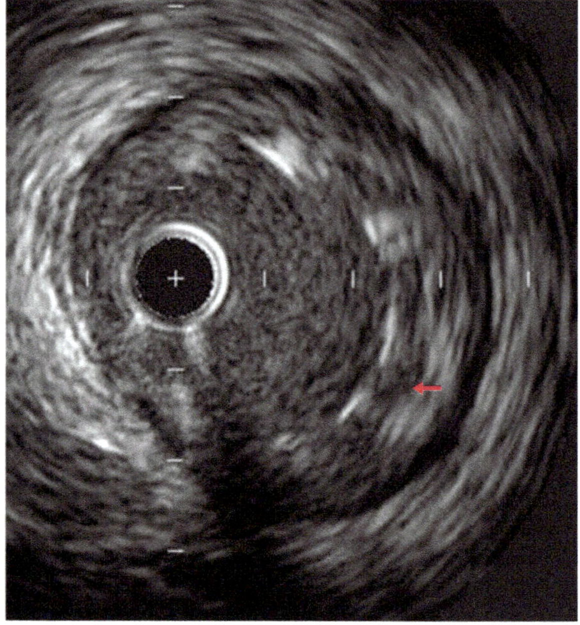

Fig. 9 Incomplete stent apposition after stent implantation. Free space can be seen between the stent struts and the surface of the intima (red arrow)

Perivascular Landmarks and Coronary Orientation for PCI

Eiji Noguchi and Yuji Oikawa

Points for Comprehensive Utilization

- A three-dimensional orientation combining coronary angiography (CAG) and IVUS findings is necessary.
- Observe the location and characteristics of the lesion as well as the direction of anterior and posterior merging branches and perivascular structures.
- We have to be aware of the direction of the epicardium and avoid risks such as vascular perforation or cardiac tamponade due to debulking or dilation of the lesion.

IVUS directly visualizes the lumen, vessel wall, and lesion of coronary arteries, and is widely used for device selection and endpoint determination during percutaneous coronary intervention (PCI). To safely and appropriately perform PCI, IVUS should be recorded after understanding CAG findings and observing the location and nature of the lesion, the direction of the plaque as well as branches that is depicted proximal and distal to the lesion.

In particular, confirmation of branches and plaque orientation is most important in directional coronary atherectomy (DCA), which was revived in 2015. Combined orientation from cross-sectional IVUS images as well as CAG with lumen silhouettes viewed in various projections are necessary.

E. Noguchi (✉)
ME Office, The Cardiovascular Institute Hospital, Minato-ku, Tokyo, Japan
e-mail: nouguchi@cvi.or.jp

Y. Oikawa
The Cardiovascular Institute Hospital, Minato-ku, Tokyo, Japan

J. Honye (ed.), *Basics of Comprehensive IVUS-Guided PCI*,
https://doi.org/10.1007/978-981-19-5658-4_5

In this section, we describe the anatomy of coronary arteries and landmarks outside the vessel that are necessary for reading IVUS and outline the importance to understand the direction of coronary plaque in relation to branches and other objects.

1 Key Points of IVUS Observation

IVUS images demonstrate a cross-section of the vessel from proximal to distal segments. The key to orienting the coronary artery is to determine the pericardial direction. Because pericardium is composed of fibrous tissue, it is depicted as a high echoic structure on IVUS (Fig. 1). However, even when recording from distal segments of the coronary artery, the pericardium may not be visualized when it is distant from the coronary artery or when the vessel diameter is large. When there are no landmarks such as branches and the direction of the pericardium is to be confirmed, the depth and gain of the device should be changed for observation.

Next, the direction of plaque localization should be confirmed after determining the direction of branches and the location of coronary veins.

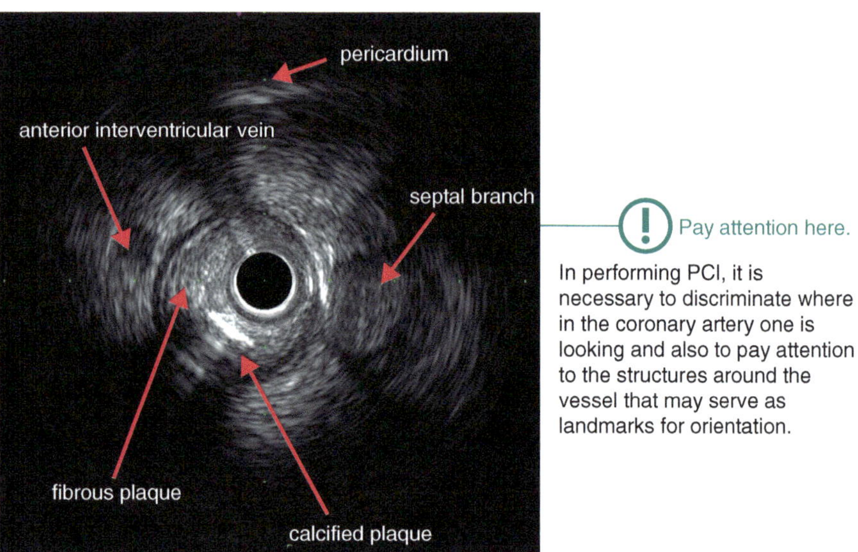

Fig. 1 IVUS image of LAD. IVUS can visualize fine structures in the coronary arteries with high resolution and can also observe extravascular structures. Pay attention here. In performing PCI, it is necessary to discriminate where in the coronary artery one is looking and also to pay attention to the structures around the vessel that may serve as landmarks for orientation

2 Coronary Anatomy and IVUS

2.1 *Left Anterior Descending Artery (LAD)*

When an IVUS catheter is inserted into the distal part of LAD and pulled back, several septal and diagonal branches are observed, and finally, a circumflex branch merges to form the left main trunk (LMT).

If the pericardial side is imagined at 12 o'clock, the myocardial side is 6 o'clock, diagonal branches usually at 9 o'clock, a circumflex artery at 7–8 o'clock, and the septal branches at 4–5 o'clock (Fig. 2).

Advice

The most reliable source of direction is the diagonal branch, and other branches should be used only as a reference because the direction of septal branches or a circumflex artery is variable. Once the diagonal branch is identified, its 90° clockwise direction is usually pericardial direction, which is often equivalent to the upper side of CAG from the right anterior oblique 30°projection.

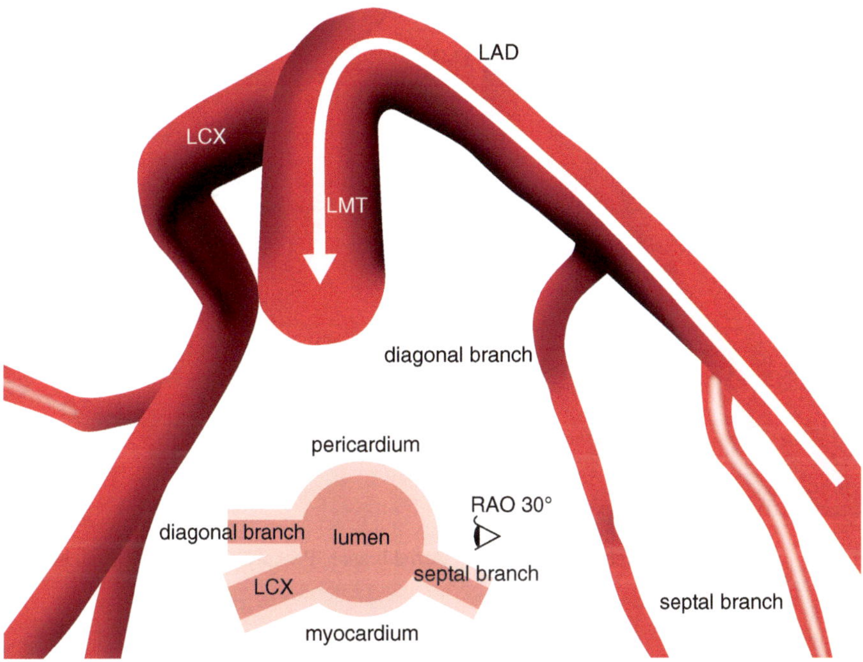

Fig. 2 LAD (direction of merging branches). Diagonal branch. Septal branch. Pericardium. Diagonal branch. Septal branch. Lumen. Endocardium. Myocardium. RAO 30°

However, since 12 o'clock is not always the pericardial direction in all coronary arteries on IVUS images, it is necessary to correct the angle from obtained images.

2.2 Left Circumflex Artery

When observed from the distal part of Left Circumflex Artery (LCX), a posterior lateral (PL), and an obtuse marginal (OM) branch are depicted, followed by an atrial branch and finally LAD. The LCX is curved and runs down along the inter-atrial groove.

In LCX, when the pericardium is imagined as 12 o'clock, the LAD in the 3 o'clock direction, the OM and PL in the 12–3 o'clock direction, and the atrial branch in the 9–12 o'clock direction (Fig. 3). However, there is a great deal of individual variability in branching patterns in LCX, and LCX may be difficult to isolate branches on CAG.

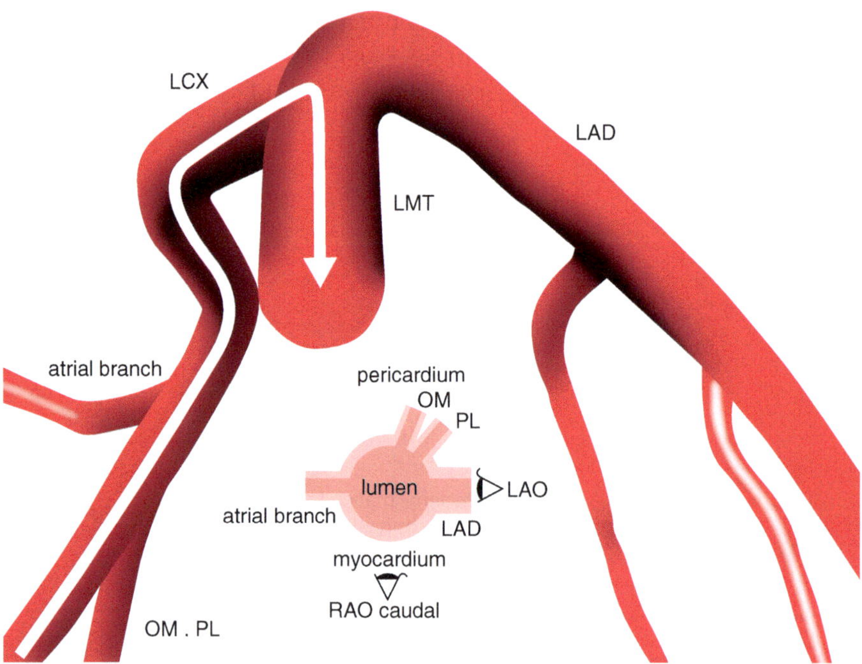

Fig. 3 LCX (merging direction of branching). Atrial branch. Pericardium. Lumen. Atrial branch. Myocardium

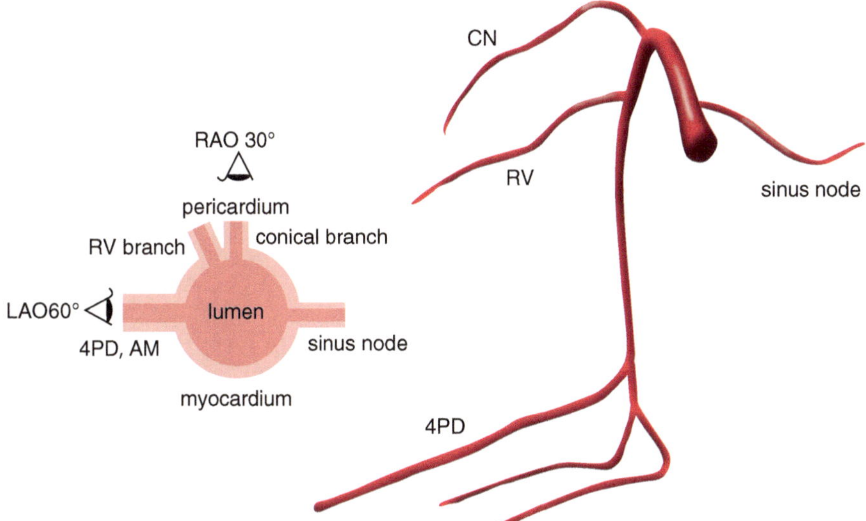

Fig. 4 Right coronary artery (direction of merging branches). Sinus node. Pericardium. Conical branch. Sinus node. Myocardium. Lumen

2.3 Right Coronary Artery

Right Coronary Artery (RCA) consists of distal seg. 4PD, an acute marginal branch (AM), a right ventricular branch (RV branch), a sinus node artery (sinus node artery), and a conus branch. When the pericardial side is imaged at 12 o'clock, IVUS images usually show the sinus node artery at 3 o'clock, the conus branch at 10–12 o'clock, the RV branch at 9–2 o'clock with large individual variation, and the seg. 4PD and acute margin branch at 8–10 o'clock (Fig. 4).

3 Perivascular Structures

3.1 Coronary Vein

During IVUS observation, perivascular structures are often seen in the vicinity of coronary arteries that do not merge, unlike branches. These are coronary veins, and they may serve as good landmarks to confirm orientation.

Coronary veins travel in several patterns, and the largest coronary vein, the great cardiac vein-coronary sinus system, is responsible for venous perfusion of the left ventricular system. The anterior interventricular vein travels along the left anterior descending artery in the anterior interventricular sulcus and gradually increases in diameter along the diagonal branch that branches from the central side to become

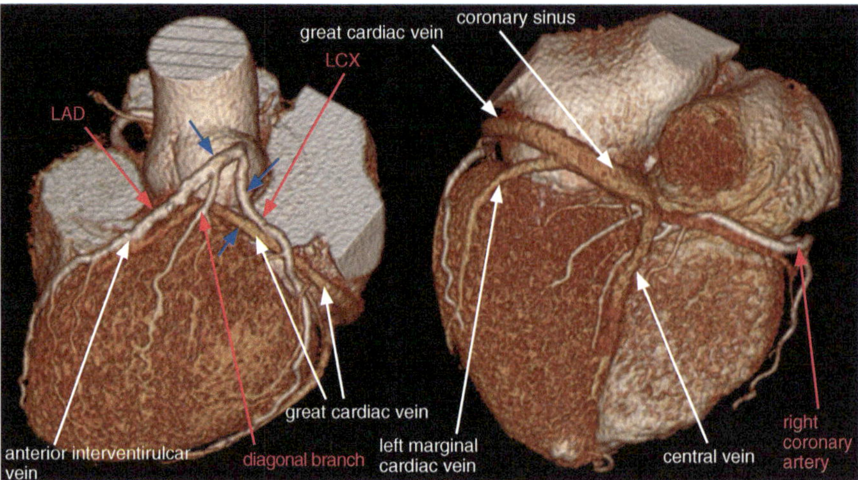

Fig. 5 Coronary artery and coronary vein travel: normal coronary artery case. Triangle of Brocq-Mouchet: The triangle is surrounded by light blue arrows (LAD, LCX, and anterior interventricular vein) in the left figure. It is called the triangle of Brocq-Mouchet. Coronary sinus. Great cardiac vein. Left circumflex. Left anterior descending branch. Anterior interventricular vein. Left marginal cardiac vein. Central vein. Great cardiac vein. Diagonal branch. Right coronary artery

continuous with the vena cava. The vena cava runs parallel to the left circumflex artery and further increases in diameter to connect to the coronary sinus (Fig. 5). Posterior interventricular veins and central veins which enter the great cardiac vein-coronary sinus system have lots of variations in numbers, sizes, and travel of venous branches. Veins involved in the right coronary artery include a small cardiac vein, which runs from the lateral to the posterior wall of the right ventricle and flows into the coronary sinus, and an anterior cardiac vein, which runs from the right atrium to the anterior wall of the right ventricle.

The anterior interventricular vein often runs on the left side of the left anterior descending artery and is often located up to 180° counterclockwise from the epicardium (Fig. 1). Veins are depicted as luminal structures with an echogenic flow that does not merge with coronary arteries.

Because the great cardiac vein runs parallel to the left circumflex artery and connects to the coronary sinus, the great cardiac vein and coronary sinus are often visualized during observation of the left circumflex artery on IVUS (Fig. 6).

The small cardiac veins and anterior cardiac veins are seen while observing the right coronary artery are depicted straddling the epicardial side, anterior to the right coronary artery such as a ladder-like appearance (Fig. 7).

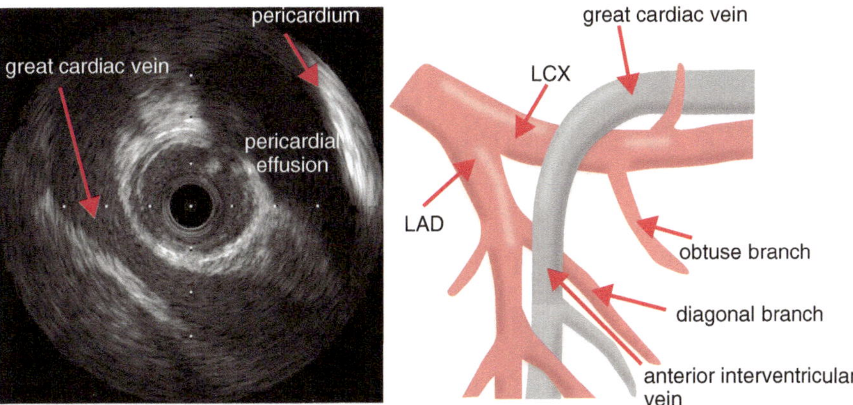

Fig. 6 Great cardiac vein. The great cardiac vein recorded from the main trunk of the LCX is shown. Because of the presence of pericardial effusion in the left panel, the pericardium was highlighted by a stronger reflection. The cardiac contraction caused the great cardiac veins to drain and collapse. Pericardium. Great cardiac vein. Pericardial effusion. Left anterior descending artery. Obtuse branch. Diagonal branch. Anterior interventricular vein. Left circumflex

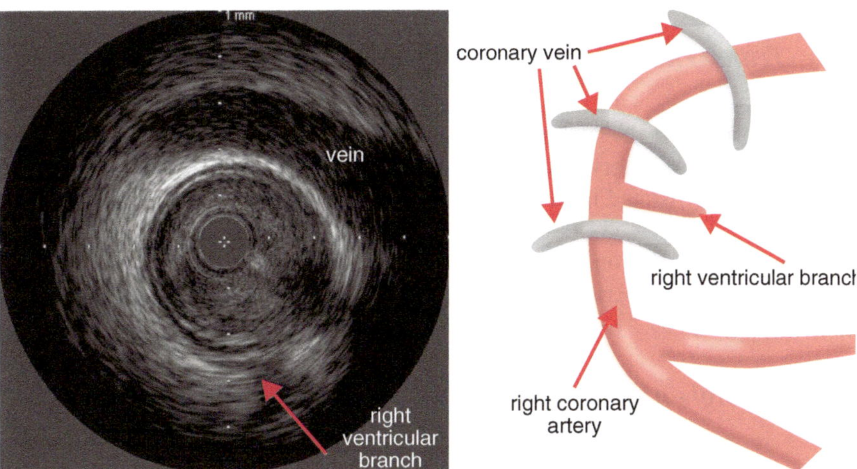

Fig. 7 Right coronary vein. The veins straddle the anterior (epicardial) side of the RCA main trunk in a ladder-like fashion, often with a right ventricular branch in their vicinity. Coronary vein. Vein. Right ventricular branch. Right ventricular branch. Right coronary artery

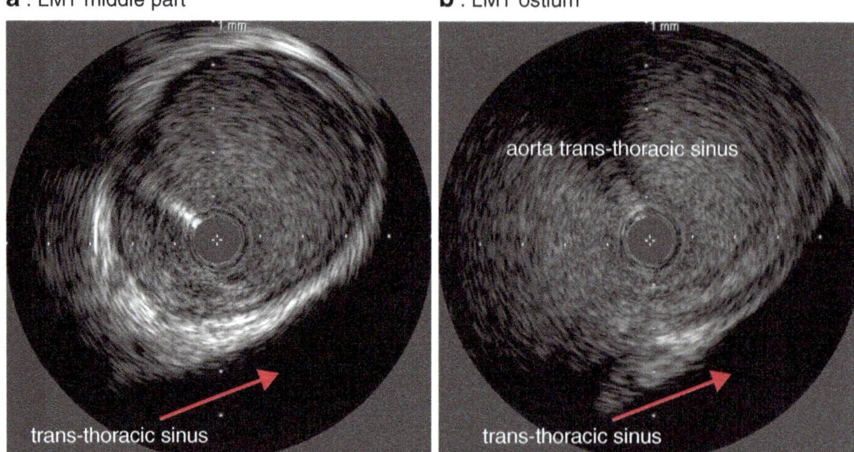

Fig. 8 Trans-thoracic sinus. The left circumflex branch joined from 12 o'clock, and as it approached the middle of the left main trunk, an anechoic space was seen from 2 to 7 o'clock. The aorta emerged from the contralateral side of the trans-thoracic sinus. (**a**) LMT middle part. (**b**) LMT ostium. Aorta trans-thoracic sinus. Middle part of left main

3.2 *Trans-Thoracic Sinus*

After pullback from the left anterior descending artery (LAD) and the confluence of the left circumflex artery (LCX), echo-free space may be seen outside the LMT (Fig. 8). This is located in the epicardial direction rotated 90° clockwise from the proximal part of merged LCX. This structure is called the trans-thoracic sinus, and it is a pericardial effusion in the area surrounded by the pericardium at the transition from the aorta to the pericardium.

3.3 *Triangle of Brocq-Mouchet*

In the proximal part of the LAD, a triangular anechoic area may be seen outside the vessel near the confluence of LCX. This is a physiological pericardial effusion surrounded by the LAD, the LCX, and the anterior interventricular vein, and is called the triangle of Brocq-Mouchet (Figs. 5 and 9).

3.4 *Myocardial Bridge*

When a coronary artery runs beneath the myocardium around the middle of LAD, functional stenosis due to cardiac contraction, called squeezing on CAG may occur. The myocardial tissue that covers a portion of this coronary artery is called a myocardial bridge (Fig. 10). An extravascular myocardial bundle runs over the coronary artery.

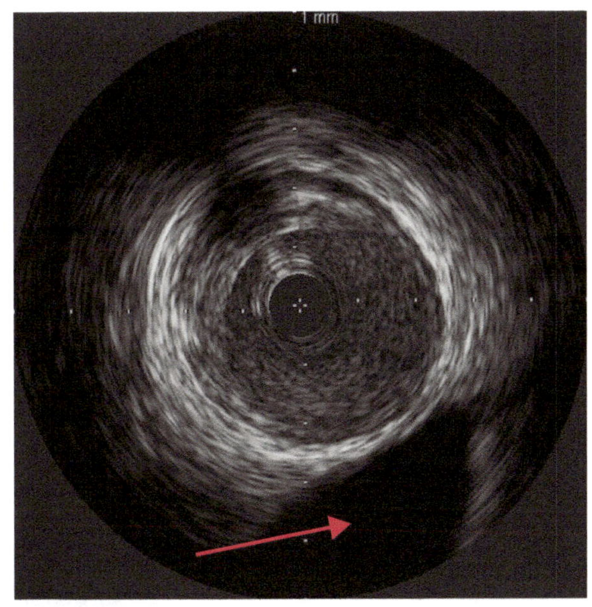

Fig. 9 Triangle of Brocq-Mouchet. A pullback from the proximal LAD may reveal a physiologic pericardial effusion area bounded by the LAD, LCX, and anterior interventricular vein delineated on the same side as the LCX

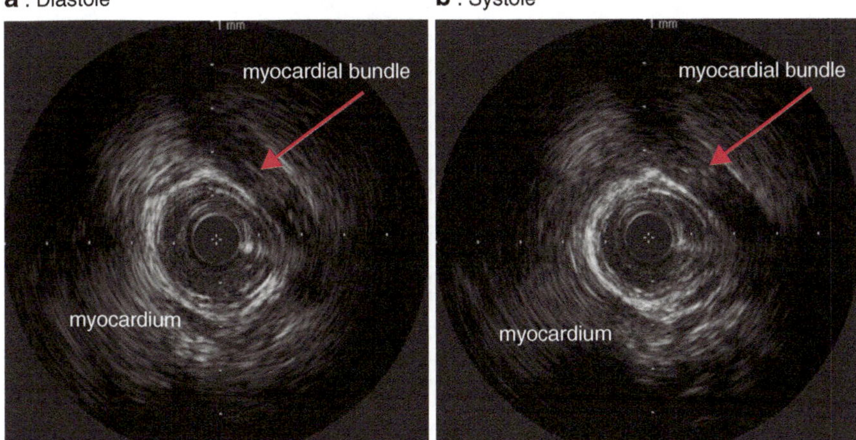

Fig. 10 Myocardial bridge. A case with mild squeezing. In typical cases, the lumen is clearly narrowed during systole and the intimal thickening may be seen. (**a**) Diastole. (**b**) Systole. Myocardial bundle. Myocardium

4 Utilize Convenient Features Equipped on the IVUS System

Terumo'ss VISICUBE® has a useful feature called multi-drive mode, which allows the operating frequency to be changed.

During the use of 60 MHz AltaView®, it is possible to select either 40 or 60 MHz (Table 1). With this feature, the resolution and penetrating depth can be adjusted for better image quality, making it possible to treat different-sized vessels, such as PCI and EVT, with a single IVUS catheter.

A case study is presented in Fig. 11.

EVT: Endovascular treatment

Table 1 Frequency of each drive mode according to catheter used

	Acoustic operating frequency	
Drive mode	AltaView®	ViewIT®/Navifocus® WR
C mode	Approx. 40 MHz	Approx. 35 MHz
E mode	Approx. 43 MHz	Approx. 38 MHz
F mode	Approx. 47 MHz	Approx. 43 MHz
G mode	Approx. 50 MHz	Approx. 44 MHz
H mode	Approx. 60 MHz	Approx. 46 MHz

Coarse; Resolution; Fine; Depth; Shallow

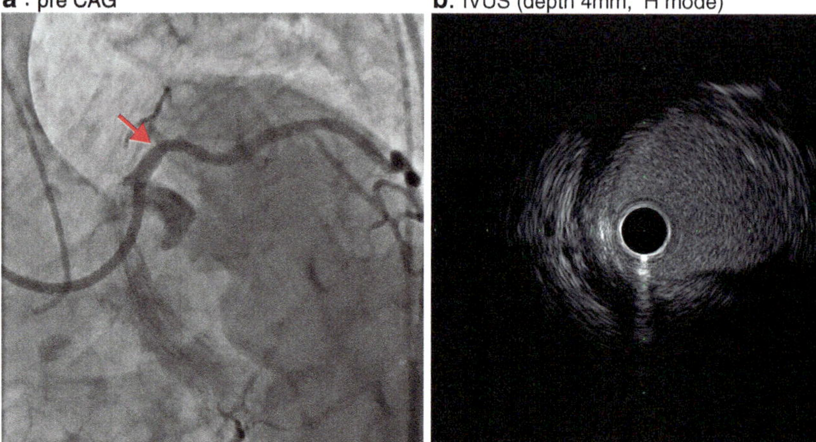

Fig. 11 IVUS-guided wiring: Case: LAD (CTO) IVUS guide wiring. (**a**) Pre–CAG. Chronic total occlusion (CTO) at the ostial LAD. (**b**) IVUS (depth 4 mm, H mode). A floppy wire was inserted into the side branch (LCx), and the ostium of the LAD was confirmed by IVUS (AltaView®) (→). (**c**) IVUS (depth 6 mm, H mode). Changed depth to 6 mm to observe a deeper area. (**d**) IVUS-guided wiring. Anterior approach under Crusade (Kaneka Corporation) support. We started with Gaia (manufactured by Asahi Intec) first, then Gaia Second, and finally Conquest Pro (manufactured by Asahi Intec), and succeeded in penetrating the entry. (**e**) IVUS (depth 6 mm, F mode). IVUS confirmed that Conquest Pro merged from the CTO. c and depth were the same, but the drive mode was changed to F (47 MHz). The image was a little rough because of the lower frequency, but the penetration depth was increased and the whole vessel image could be understood. (**f**) Final CAG. Final angiography

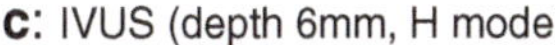
c: IVUS (depth 6mm, H mode)

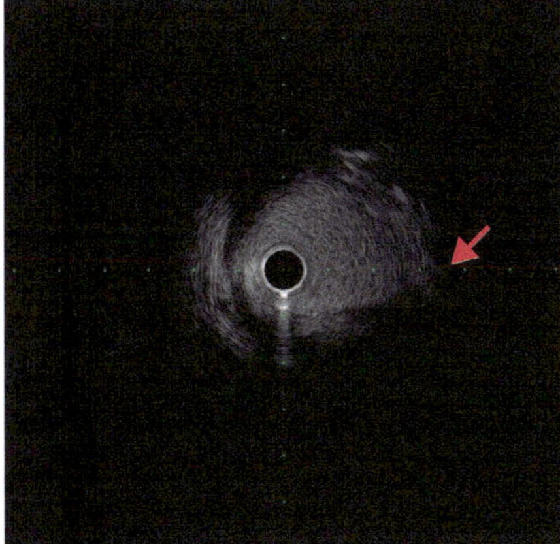

Changed depth to 6mm to observe a deeper area. Ostial LAD (→)

d: IVUS-guided wiring

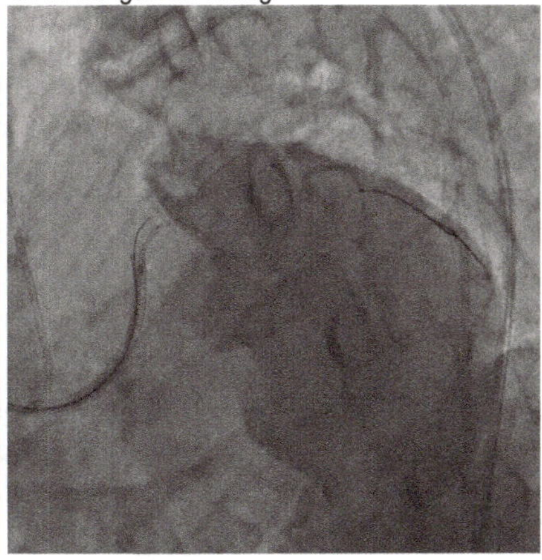

Anterior approach under Crusade (Kaneka Corporation) support. We started with Gaia (manufactured by Asahi Intec) first, then Gaia Second, and finally Conquest Pro (manufactured by Asahi Intec), and succeeded in penetrating the entry.

e: IVUS (depth 6mm, F mode)

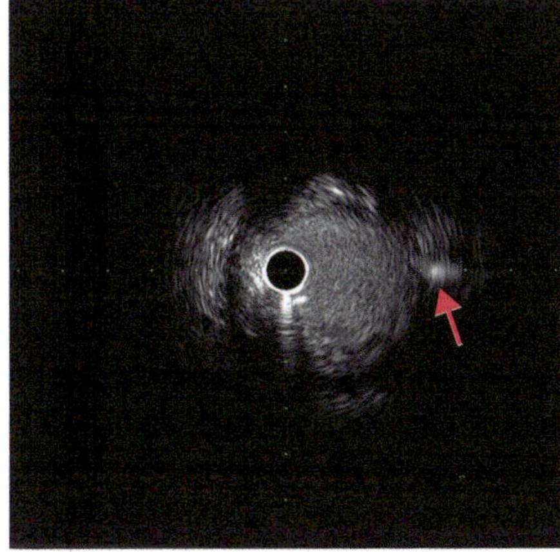

IVUS confirmed that Conquest Pro merged from the CTO. c and depth were the same, but the drive mode was changed to F (47MHz). The image was a little rough because of the lower frequency, but the penetration depth was increased and the whole vessel image could be understood.

f: final CAG

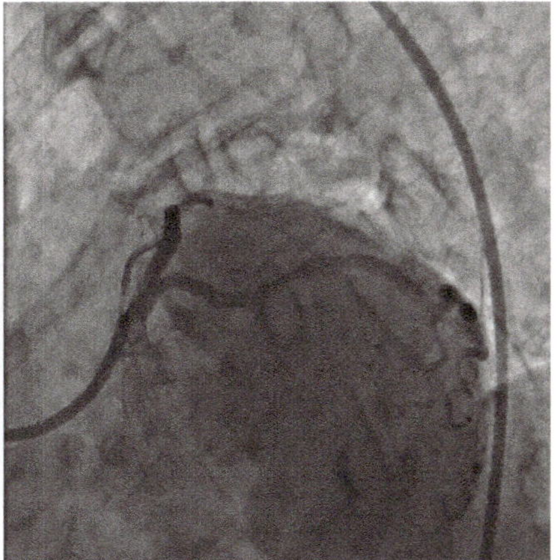

final angiography

Fig. 11 (continued)

5 To Perform IVUS-Guided PCI Effectively and Safely

In order to decide strategies for treatment, the direction of the plaque must first be determined. Landmarks such as epicardium, bifurcations, coronary veins, and myocardial bridges can be used for this purpose.

6 Pay Attention Here

When a large amount of calcified or fibrous plaque is on the myocardial side in eccentric lesions, there is a risk of cardiac tamponade due to vessel perforation following lesion dilation so that operators should carefully select balloon or stent size with adequate inflation pressure.

Lesions for which DCA will be used in the future include bifurcation lesions such as the distal left main trunk, bifurcation lesions with LAD and LCX or lesions in the middle portion with large branches, as well as lesions in the proximal and middle right coronary artery, all of which require identification of epicardial direction and IVUS guidance is mandatory.

We would like to continue to make full use of IVUS to provide safe and effective treatment.

Suggested Readings

Honye J, Saito S. IVUS manual. Nakayama Shoten: Tokyo; 2006. p. 39–47.
Oikawa Y. PCI from now on. Tokyo: Medical View; 2013. p. 82–90.
Sumitsuji S, Nakatani A. IVUS & logical intervention. Tokyo: Medical Sense; 2004. p. 85–127.
Yajima J. Cardiac catheterization from now on. Tokyo: Medical View; 2013. p. 315–27.

Understand the Dilatation Mechanism of PCI

Atsuko Kodama and Mitsuyasu Terashima

Points for Comprehensive Utilization

- Morphology and characteristics of the plaque (eccentric or concentric, presence of calcium or lipid core, attenuated plaque) should be interpreted from IVUS.
- Based on the IVUS findings, the dilatation mechanism of the lesion and a site of dissection following dilatation should be predicted.
- The optimal strategy for PCI is then determined, and safe and effective PCI should be performed.

Currently, IVUS is an indispensable device for PCI. IVUS provides information on the distribution, morphology, and characteristics of the plaque, which can be used to select an optimal device for PCI. In addition, operators can understand high-risk lesions that may cause serious complications such as coronary perforation, and prevent them based on IVUS findings.

In order to fully utilize the information from IVUS, understanding the mechanism of coronary lumen dilatation by balloons and stents and speculating on the dilatation mechanism for each lesion will enable safer and more effective PCI.

A. Kodama · M. Terashima (✉)
Department of Cardiology, Toyohashi Heart Center, Toyohashi, Aichi, Japan
e-mail: terashima@heart-center.or.jp

J. Honye (ed.), *Basics of Comprehensive IVUS-Guided PCI*,
https://doi.org/10.1007/978-981-19-5658-4_6

1 Mechanism of Coronary Lumen Dilation

The mechanism of dilatation by balloons and stents is mainly due to 1. vessel stretch and 2. plaque redistribution in the long axis. Depending on the characteristics of the plaque, 3. spillage of the plaque contents due to mechanical disruption of the plaque may also contribute to vessel dilatation. The combination of these factors dilates the coronary artery lumen, but the percentage of contribution varies depending on the characteristics of the plaque. In cases with directional coronary atherectomy (DCA), the lumen expands due to both 1. vessel stretch and 4. debulking of plaque.

2 Vessel Stretch

When vessel stretch occurs, plaque dissection generally occurs. When radial force is applied to the plaque by balloon dilatation, it first expands from the thinnest part of the plaque (Fig. 1b). Then, tears appear at both ends of the thick plaque (plaque shoulder), and dissection occurs from the lumen to the media (Fig. 1c). At the site

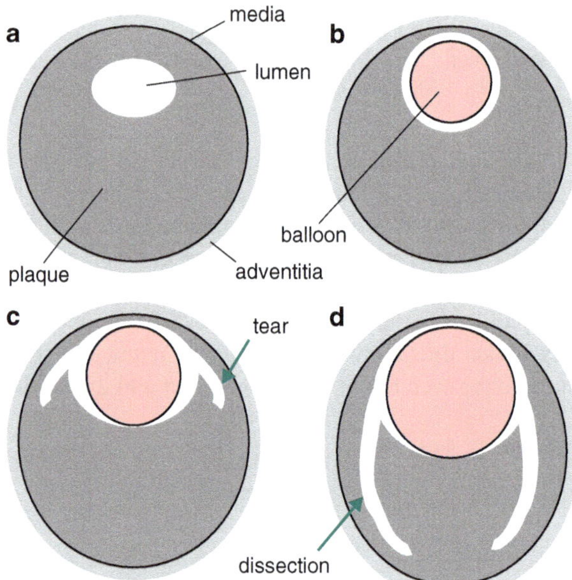

Fig. 1 Vessel stretch ([1] Ueno K: Coronary Intervention 2004, modified in part). (**a**) Plaque is thinnest at 12 o'clock and thickest at 6 o'clock. (**b**) When radial force is applied by balloon dilatation, it first expands from the 12 o'clock direction, where the plaque is the thinnest. (**c**) Dissection is subsequently formed by cracks at both ends of the thicker portion of the plaque. At the site of dissection, the plaque separates and the lumen widens as its outer wall expands. (**d**) With additional radial force, the dissociation proceeds to depth. Media, lumen, plaque, outer membrane, balloon, crack, dissection

of dissection, the plaque separates and its outer wall expands to enlarge the lumen. If the radial force continues to be applied, the crack extends to the deeper part of the plaque, creating a large dissection (Fig. 1d) [2].

These reactions are more likely to occur in eccentric plaques because dissection tends to occur at the border between thin and thick plaques. In calcified lesions, dissection tends to occur at the edge of the calcium and often forms a large dissection behind calcium.

According to the IVUS study by Honye et al., plaque morphology after balloon dilatation is classified into the following six types according to the morphology of dissection [3].

Type A: Linear tear toward the media, not reaching the media (Fig. 2).

Type B: Dissection involving the media with no dissection behind the plaque (Fig. 3).

Type C: Dissection behind the plaque up to 180° (Fig. 4).

Type D: 180°–360° dissection behind the plaque (Fig. 5).

Type E: Plaque extension but no tear or dissection.

Type E_1: In a concentric plaque (Fig. 6a)

Type E_2: In an eccentric plaque (Fig. 6b)

In this report, eccentric plaques were found in 73% of IVUS lesions, and 77% of them had tears or dissection, whereas only 22% of concentric plaques had tears or dissection. In addition, 66% of calcified lesions had tears or dissection, whereas only 25% of non-calcified lesions had tears or dissection. After balloon dilatation, there was no significant difference in area % stenosis on IVUS between the types, but restenosis rate within 6 months was seen in 50% of Type E1 lesions, which was significantly higher than the average of 12% for the other types ($p = 0.053$).

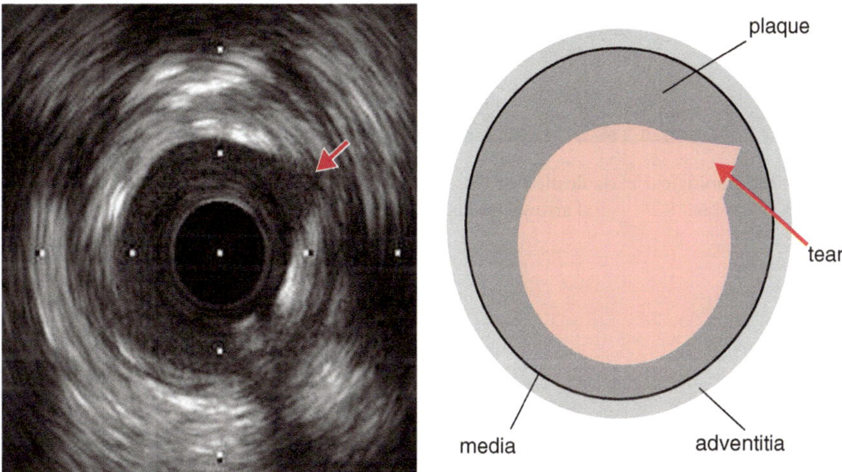

Fig. 2 Morphological classification of dissection Type A. A tear toward the media is seen at 2 o'clock (→). It does not reach the media. Plaque, tear, adventitia, media

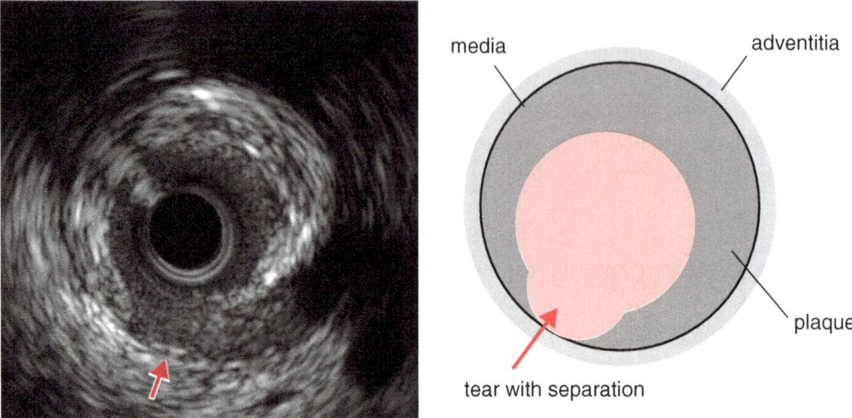

Fig. 3 Morphological classification of dissection Type B. Dissection extending into the media at 7 o'clock (→). There is no dissection behind the plaque (Tear with separation)

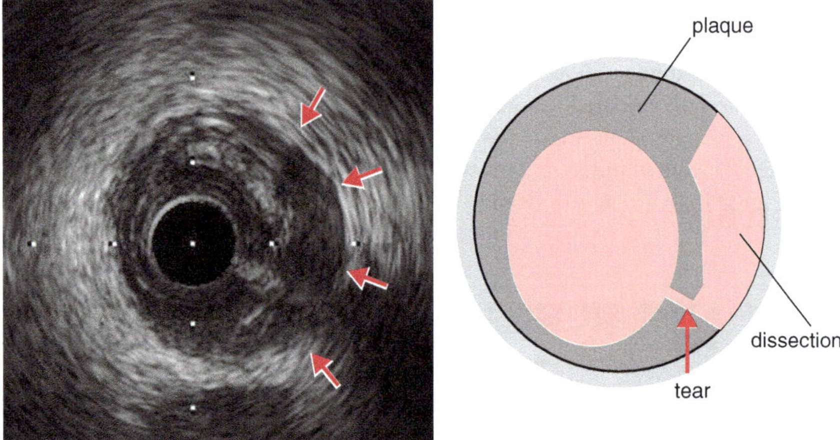

Fig. 4 Morphological classification of dissection Type C. Dissociation is observed from 2 to 5 o'clock over about 90° (→ red arrow). Plaque, dissection, crack

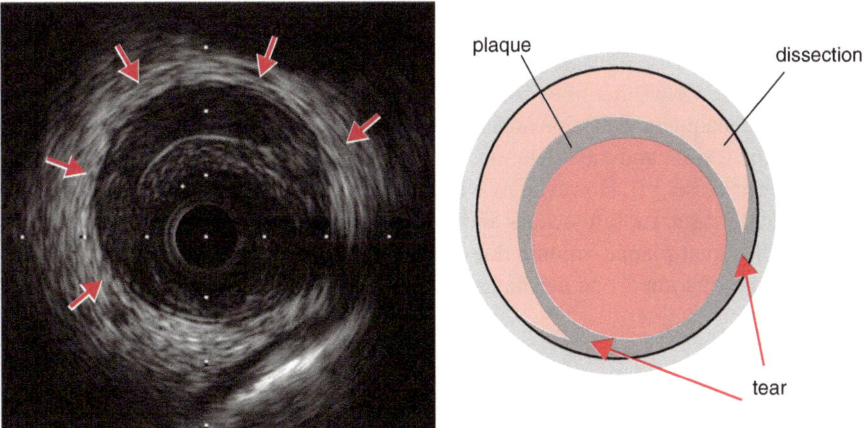

Fig. 5 Morphological classification of dissection Type D. Dissection is observed from 7 o'clock to 3 o'clock, over about 240° (→). Plaque, dissection, crack

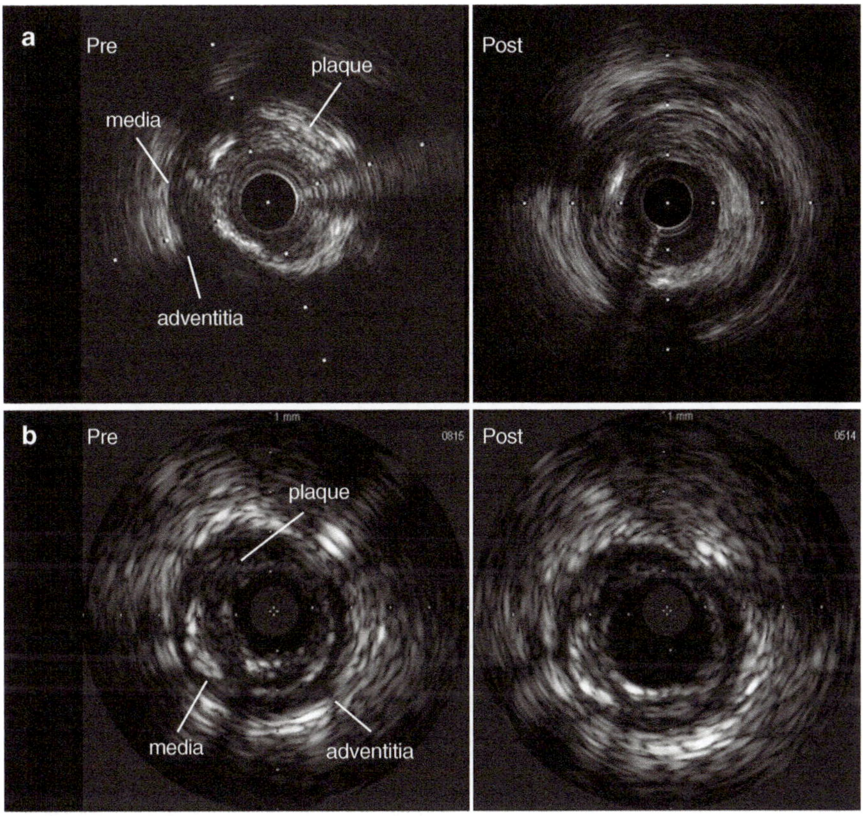

Fig. 6 Morphological classification of dissection Type E. (**a**) Type E_1. Concentric plaque is present. Extension of the plaque is seen with balloon dilatation, but no tear or dissection is seen. (**b**) Type E_2. Eccentric plaque is present. Extension of the plaque is seen with balloon dilatation, but no tear or dissection is seen. Plaque, media, adventitia

3 Plaque Redistribution in the Longitudinal Direction

Mintz et al. reported that after balloon dilatation, the total plaque volume did not change, the plaque in the lesion area shifted to the reference vessel site proximal and distal to the lesion, and the dilatation of the lumen was mainly due to the dilatation of the entire vessel [4]. However, as will be described later, there are cases in which mechanical plaque rupture occurs and the contents flow out, and it is questionable whether the total plaque volume does not change, but it is clear that longitudinal plaque redistribution is one mechanism of lumen dilatation.

4 Mechanical Plaque Disruption

In lesions with large lipid cores, such as acute coronary syndromes, plaque volume is reduced by the outflow of plaque content due to mechanical plaque disruption, which is considered to be one of the mechanisms of coronary lumen dilation.

Prati et al. found that vessel stretch and mechanical plaque disruption contributed to 87% and 13%, respectively, unstable angina, whereas vessel stretch and mechanical plaque disruption contributed to 47% and 53%, respectively, in unstable angina ($p < 0.05$) [5].

5 Debulking

The atheroma is directly removed by DCA, which leads to a significant decrease in plaque in the lesion. However, the device is large and causes some vessel stretching. It is reported that 76% of the lumen enlargement was due to plaque reduction and 24% was due to vessel stretching [6, 7].

6 Understanding Dilatation Mechanisms and Its Application to PCI

By evaluating plaque morphology and characteristics such as eccentricity, calcification, lipid core, and attenuated plaque, by IVUS, the mechanism of lesion dilatation and the site of dissection after dilatation can be estimated to some extent. By combining this information with the "lumen diameter at the reference vessel site" and "vessel diameter at the lesion site," it is possible to determine the balloon/stent size that will provide sufficient dilation to allow for therapeutic dissection. The stent size can be determined.

Pay Attention Here

In cases of severe calcification, conventional balloons or stents may not be able to dilate the lesions sufficiently. Therefore, alternative methods such as scoring balloons or a rotablator should be taken into account.

Knowing the mechanism of dilatation can also help prevent complications. In the case of an eccentric plaque with hard parts on the plaque side, such as superficial calcification or hard fibrous plaque, the expansion pressure by the balloon or stent is concentrated on the softer areas of the vessel wall, which can lead to coronary perforation as a serious complication (Fig. 7). In such lesions with extremely uneven vessel wall stiffness, it is necessary to use IVUS information to prevent perforation.

Advice

For example, it is useful to use a rotablator if ablation is possible while paying attention to wire bias. If ablation is difficult, it is important to select a balloon with a smaller size, apply pressure gradually while checking IVUS, and gradually increase the size of the balloon if necessary to ensure adequate predilation before stent placement.

There is a higher risk of coronary artery perforation if the balloon or stent size is large (balloon/vessel diameter ratio greater than 1.3) or if burr size of rotablator is large (burr/vessel diameter ratio greater than 0.8).

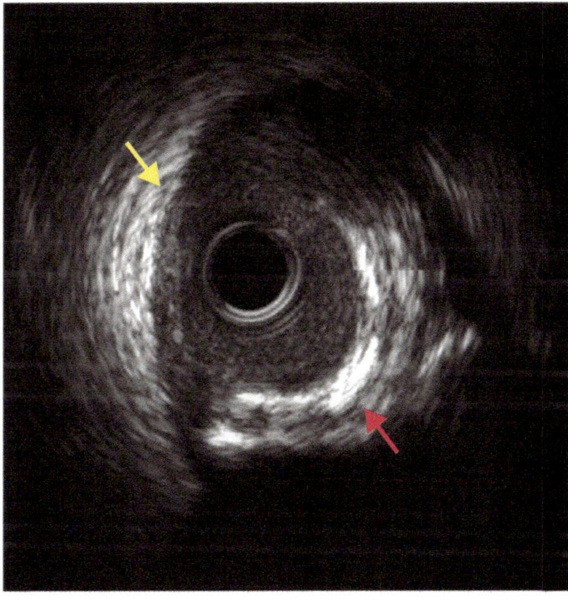

Fig. 7 High-risk lesions for coronary artery perforation. An eccentric plaque is seen in the 2–7 o'clock direction with superficial calcification (→ red arrow). There is no plaque on the opposite side (=> yellow arrow)

To improve PCI outcomes and safety, it is important to understand the mechanism of coronary lumen dilation by balloons, stents, and DCA. IVUS can help us perform PCI correctly and reliably.

References

1. Ueno K, Awachi Y, Hattori A. IVUS-guided POBA. Coronary Intervention. 2004;3:56–61.
2. Block PC, Myler RK, Stertzer S, et al. Morphology after transluminal angioplasty in human beings. N Engl J Med. 1981;305:382–5.
3. Honye J, Donald JM, Ashit J, et al. Morphological effects of coronary balloon angioplasty in vivo assessment by intravascular ultrasound imaging. Circulation. 1992;85:1012–25.
4. Mintz G, Pichard A, Kent K, et al. Axial plaque redistribution as a mechanism of percutaneous transluminal coronary angioplasty. Am J Cardiol. 1996;77:427–30.
5. Prati F, Pawlowski T, Gil R, et al. Stenting of culprit lesion in unstable angina leads to a marked reduction in plaque burden: a major role of plaque A serial intravascular ultrasound study. Circulation. 2003;107:2320–5.
6. Takeda Y, Tsuchikane E, Kobayashi T, et al. Effects of plaque debulking before stent implantation on in-stent neointimal proliferation: a serial 3-dimensional intravascular ultrasound study. Am Heart J. 2003;146:175–82.
7. Suzuki T, Hosokawa H, Katoh O, et al. Effects of adjunctive balloon angioplasty after intravascular ultrasound-guided optimal directional coronary. J Am Coll Cardiol. 1999;34:1028–35.

Can IVUS be Used as an Indicator of Ischemia?

Shoichi Kuramitsu

Points for Comprehensive Utilization

- The cutoff value for minimum lumen area (MLA) depends on the target vessel diameter, but 3.0 mm^2 is recommended for non-left main lesions.
- The diagnostic performance of ischemia can be improved by adding % area stenosis >60% to MLA.
- IVUS is useful for evaluating ischemia in left coronary main trunk (LMCA) lesions, and MLA <4.5 mm^2 indicates ischemia, and MLA >6.0 mm^2 indicates no ischemia.

1 Relationship Between MLA and FFR

Fractional flow reserve (FFR) is a well-established method for assessing ischemia in coronary artery lesions. The 2018 ESC guidelines recommend it as Class I for the ischemic assessment of coronary moderate stenosis lesions. On the other hand, IVUS is recommended as Class IIa for assessing the functional severity of non-protective LMCA lesions but not for other lesions [1]. Therefore, FFR is generally used to diagnose ischemia in moderately stenotic lesions in clinical practice, and IVUS-guided percutaneous coronary intervention (PCI) is performed if ischemia is present. However, when performing PCI for tandem or diffuse lesions with severe stenosis, we often face difficulty using FFR and IVUS, mainly due to national insurance limitations. We should decide the PCI strategy based on IVUS findings in such a situation.

S. Kuramitsu (✉)
Sapporo Cardio Vascular Clinic, Sapporo, Hokkaido, Japan
e-mail: kuramitsu@heart-kizuna.com

J. Honye (ed.), *Basics of Comprehensive IVUS-Guided PCI*,
https://doi.org/10.1007/978-981-19-5658-4_7

2 Relationship Between IVUS and FFR

Bernoulli's simplified equation is helpful to understand the relationship between IVUS and FFR. In this equation, the relationship between pressure and blood flow in fluid stenosis is shown as "$\Delta P = L \times V2/A$ (ΔP: pressure gradient, L: lesion length, V: blood flow, A: luminal cross-sectional area)". Given that ΔP is equivalent to FFR, it would be possible to determine ischemia by IVUS-MLA. The meta-analysis studies have reported the relationship between IVUS-MLA and FFR (Tables 1 and 2) [2]. In the FIRST study, the only multicenter prospective study to examine the relationship between IVUS and FFR, the cutoff value was determined according to the reference vessel diameter (RVD), and the overall cutoff value was 3.07 mm^2, 2.4 mm^2 for vessels <3.0 mm, 2.7 mm^2 for vessels 3.0–3.5 mm, and 3.6 mm^2 for vessels ≥3.5 mm (Fig. 1) [3]. As such, the MLA cutoff value varies depending on the vessel diameter, but in any case, the sensitivity and specificity are about 60–70% and AUC 0.78–0.79, respectively, and the diagnosis of ischemia by MLA seems not clinically sufficient.

Table 1 Relationship between IVUS-MLA and FFR in non-LMCA lesions (modified from Refs. [2, 3])

Test	Number of lesions	FFR	MLA cutoff (mm^2)	Sensitivity (%)	Specificity (%)	AUC
Takagi et al.	51	0.75	3.0	83.0	92.3	NA
Ben-Dor et al.	92	0.80	3.2	69.2	68.3	0.73
Kang et al.	236	0.80	2.4	90.0	60.0	0.80
Waksman et al.	367	0.80	3.07	64.0	64.9	0.65

Table 2 Meta-analysis of diagnostic accuracy of FFR <0.80 by IVUS-MLA in non-LMCA lesions (modified from Ref. [2])

	Overall MLA	MLA (vessel >3 mm)	MLA (vessel <3 mm)
IVUS-MLA cutoff (mm^2)	2.36–4.0	2.4–3.2	2.4–2.59
Sensitivity	0.68 (0.65–0.71)	0.78 (0.72–0.83)	0.68 (0.62–0.74)
Specificity	0.68 (0.66–0.70)	0.66 (0.62–0.70)	0.73 (0.69–0.77)
Positive likelihood ratio	2.40 (1.90–3.10)	2.70 (2.30–3.10)	2.65 (2.45–4.30)
Negative likelihood ratio	0.30 (0.20–0.50)	0.26 (0.20–0.35)	0.27 (0.24–0.31)
AUC	0.78 (0.73–0.84)	0.78 (0.73–0.84)	0.79 (0.70–0.89)

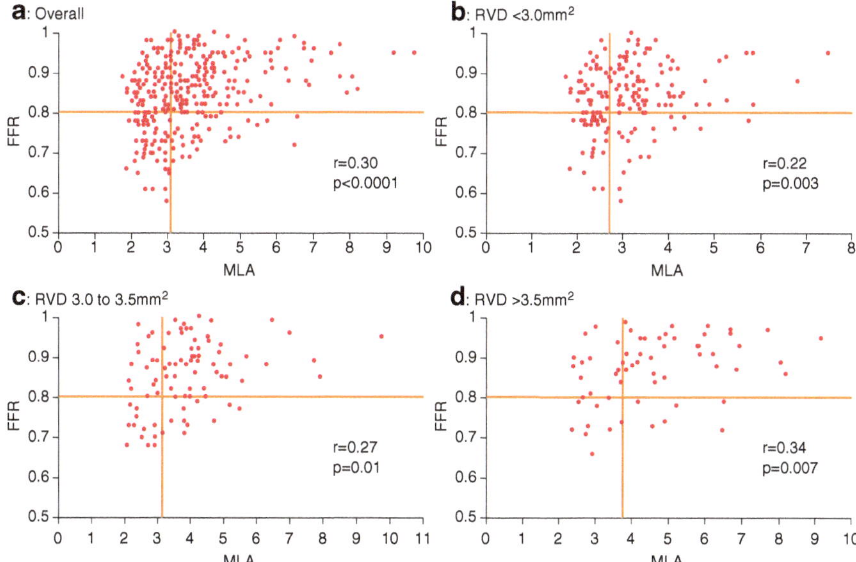

Fig. 1 Relationship between MLA and FFR. The cutoff value for MLA differs according to the reference vessel diameter (RVD) (modified from Ref. [2]). (**a**) Overall. (**b**) RVD < 3.0 mm^2. (**c**) RVD 3.0–3.5 mm^2. (**d**) RVD >3.5 mm^2

3 How to Improve the Ischemic Diagnostic Performance of IVUS?

In order to improve the diagnostic performance of IVUS for ischemia, the combination of multiple IVUS indices has been attempted. Cho et al. examined the relationship between three indices of IVUS (MLA, %plaque burden, and combination of these two indices) and FFR ≤0.80 and reported the best cutoff values for MLA and %plaque burden were 3.0 mm^2 and >75%, respectively. However, since each diagnostic performance was low with AUCs of 0.618, 0.511, and 0.516, the composite index of IVUS did not improve ischemia diagnosis [4]. This study also investigated the cause of discordance between IVUS indices and FFR findings. As non-left anterior descending (LAD) lesions were identified as predictors for mismatch (MLA ≤3.0 mm^2 and %plaque burden >75% but FFR >0.80), it is interesting that LAD lesions were identified as predictors for reverse mismatch (MLA >3.0 mm^2 and %plaque burden ≤75% but FFR ≤0.80) (Table 3).

The most crucial factor in Bernoulli's simplified equation is blood flow because blood flow is proportional to the amount of perfused myocardium, and blood flow is faster in LAD than in non-LAD. This physiological mechanism is related to the predictors of mismatch and reverses mismatch, and the lesion site should be considered when determining ischemia by IVUS. On the other hand, Takagi et al. reported that all lesions meeting both MLA <3.0 mm^2 and %area stenosis (relative stenosis)

Table 3 Factors associated with discordance between IVUS findings and FFR values (modified from Ref. [4])

	Odds ratio	95% CI	*p*-value
Predictors of mismatch			
Non-LAD lesion	2.44	1.62–3.69	<0.001
Predictors of reverse mismatch			
LAD lesion	2.68	1.71–4.19	<0.001
Race (Asian)	0.39	0.22–0.70	0.001
Left ventricular systolic function	0.98	0.96–0.99	0.0023

CI confidence intervals

>60% had an FFR <0.75 [5]. The %area stenosis is an index that considers the diameter of the target vessel, suggesting that the combination of %area stenosis and MLA may improve the diagnostic performance of IVUS for ischemia.

Pay Attention Here
The MLA naturally varies depending on the diameter of the target vessel. In addition, myocardial ischemia relies not only on MLA but also on lesion location, lesion length, and myocardial perfusion volume, which limits the ability of MLA to diagnose ischemia.

4 Utilization of IVUS for Evaluation of Ischemia in LMCA Lesions

4.1 LMCA Lesions Frequently Show Reverse Mismatchs

It is not uncommon to encounter LMCA lesions with moderate stenosis in clinical practice. Even experienced cardiologists have difficulty determining whether a lesion is functionally significant based on coronary angiographic findings alone. In particular, reverse mismatch (stenosis <50% and FFR ≤0.80) is observed in approximately 40% of LMCA lesions (Fig. 2) [6]. Figure 3 shows a representative case with a reverse mismatch in the LMCA lesion. Coronary angiography showed moderate stenosis, but FFR was 0.68 at distal LAD, and IVUS-MLA was 3.7 mm^2 (Fig. 3). Since LMCA lesions are potentially lethal once an event occurs, we should carefully evaluate their ischemia based on FFR and IVUS.

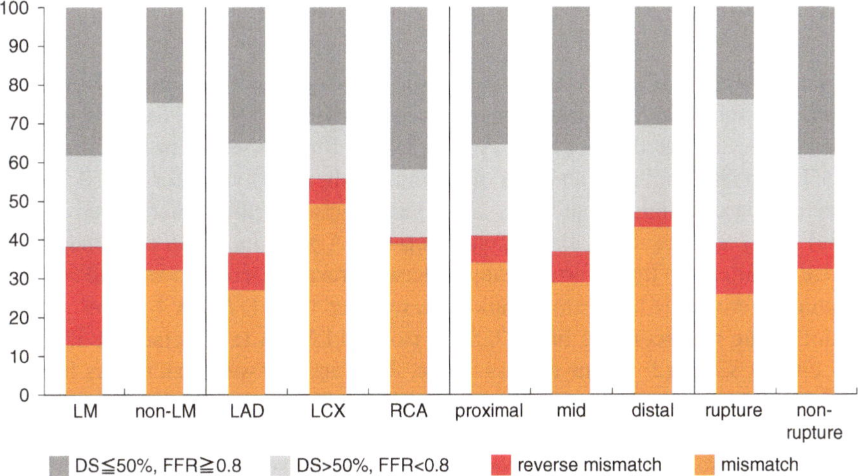

Fig. 2 Frequency of visual-functional mismatch at the lesion site. The reverse mismatch is more common in LMCA lesions and rupture sites, and mismatch is more common in LCX lesions. DS: Diameter stenosis (modified from Ref. [6]). DS ≦ 50%, FFR ≧ 0.8. DS > 50%, FFR < 0.8. Reverse mismatch, mismatch

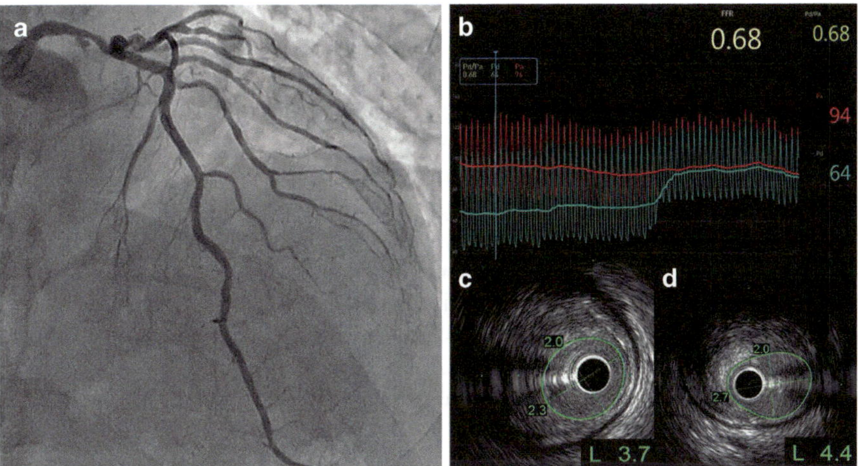

Fig. 3 A representative case of LMCA lesion with reverse mismatch. (**a**) Coronary angiography shows moderate stenosis of LMCA with plaque rupture. (**b**) FFR is 0.68 at distal LAD, and the largest step up is observed at the LMCA site. (**c** and **d**) IVUS pullback from LAD shows an MLA of 3.7 mm^2, while IVUS from LCX shows a different MLA of 4.4 mm^2

4.2 Evidence for IVUS-MLA in LMCA Lesions

Similar to non-LMCA lesions, several studies have been reported on IVUS-MLA in LMCA lesions (Table 4). Jasti et al. reported an MLA of 5.9 mm^2 (sensitivity 93%, specificity 95%) as the IVUS-MLA cutoff value for FFR <0.75 in LMCA lesions [7]. The LITRO trial used an MLA of 6.0 mm^2 as the cutoff value for LMCA lesions and compared clinical outcomes at 2 years between the Defer group (MLA >6.0 mm^2) and the revascularization group (MLA ≤6.0 mm^2). In this study, only 4.4% of patients in the deferred group underwent revascularization and had no myocardial infarction [8]. Recently, Park et al. reported that (1) MLA 4.5 mm^2 was the cutoff value for predicting FFR ≤0.80 in isolated LMCA lesions (sensitivity 77%, specificity 82%); (2) plaque rupture image, BMI, and age were risk factors for FFR ≤0.80. These results indicate that isolated LMCA lesions correlate better with FFR than non-LMCA lesions because of their relatively short lesion length, which limits the target vessel diameter and myocardial perfusion to some extent.

4.3 Difficulty in Functional Assessment of LMCA Lesions by FFR

Although FFR is useful in evaluating ischemia in LMCA lesions, physiological evaluation of the LMCA lesions can be challenging, especially in ostial stenosis or concomitant disease in LAD or left circumflex coronary artery (LCX) lesions. Recently, the J-CONFIRM Registry, which examined the clinical outcomes of Japanese patients with FFR-based deferral of revascularization, reported that LMCA lesion was associated with two-year target vessel failure [9]. In clinical practice, we experience more cases in which LMT lesions are accompanied by LAD or LCX lesions than LMT lesions alone. Therefore, comprehensive ischemic diagnosis using FFR and IVUS therapy would be ideal, but it is difficult to achieve in practice. In this regard, the EAPCI Expert Consensus suggests that it appears reasonable to defer revascularization if the IVUS-MLA is >6.0 mm^2, intervene if the IVUS-MLA <4.5 mm^2, and consider further evaluation with FFR if the IVUS-MLA is 4.5–6.0 mm^2 (Fig. 4) [11].

Table 4 Relationship between IVUS-MLA and FFR in LMCA lesions (modified from documents [2, 7, 9])

Test	Number of lesions	FFR	MLA cutoff (mm^2)	Sensitivity (%)	Specificity (%)	AUC
Jasti et al.	55	0.75	5.9	93	95	NA
Kang et al.	55	0.80	4.8	89	83	0.90
Park et al.	112	0.80	4.5	77	82	0.83

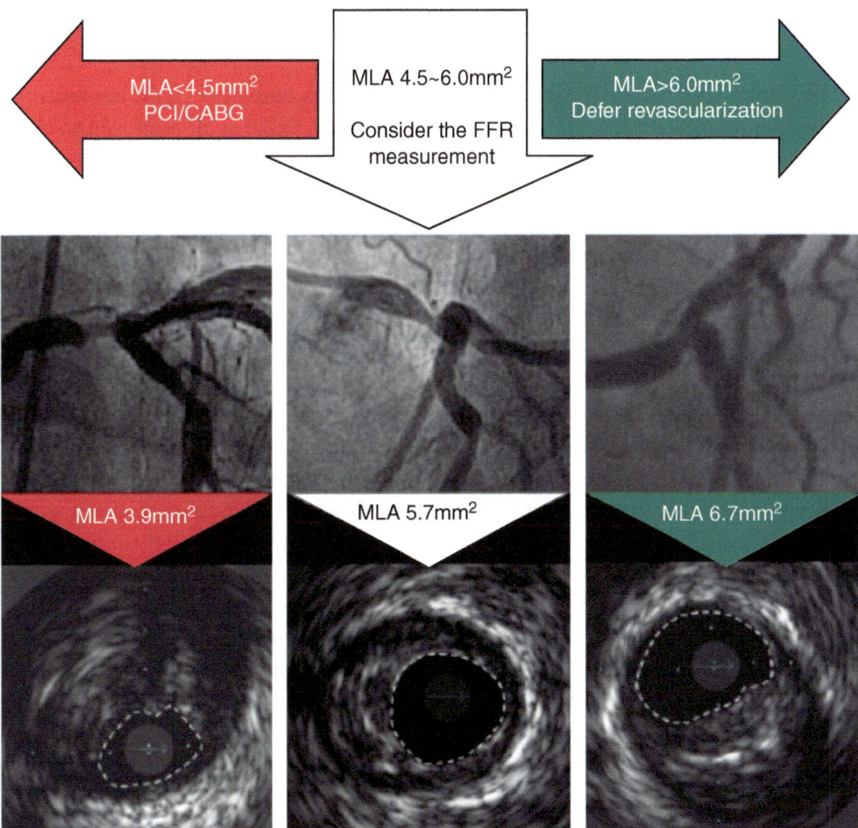

Fig. 4 Treatment strategy for LMCA lesions based on IVUS-MLA (modified from Ref. [10]). MLA < 4.5 mm^2, PCI/CABG, MLA 4.5–6.0 mm^2, consider the FFR measurement, MLA > 6.0 mm^2, Defer Defer revascularization, MLA 3.9 mm^2, MLA 5.7 mm^2, MLA 6.7 mm^2

Here's the Trick

In the case of LMCA lesions, the axis of the IVUS catheter and the vessel is likely to be misaligned (resulting in an oblique cross-section on the IVUS image), leading to an overestimation of the MLA. For accurate MLA measurement, it is essential to ensure the coaxiality of the guiding catheter and to perform IVUS pullback from both LAD and LCX.

5 A New Ischemic Index Using IVUS

As mentioned above, ischemic assessment by IVUS is based on MLA, but recently, new ischemic indices using IVUS have been reported. Seike et al. proposed an algorithm to calculate IVUS-derived FFR by incorporating data obtained from IVUS (MLA, lumen area of the reference area, and lesion length) into a simplified formula for fluid dynamics. This study retrospectively analyzed 50 lesions in 48 patients in whom IVUS and FFR were measured to compare whether IVUS-derived FFR or IVUS-MLA correlated better with FFR. As a result, IVUS-derived FFR showed a strong correlation with FFR ($R = 0.78$, $p < 0.001$) and was superior to IVUS-MLA ($R = 0.43$, $ss = 0.002$) [12]. Takami et al. reported that IB-IVUS (integrated backscatter IVUS) could predict FFR ≤0.75 more accurately than IVUS-MLA by measuring ΔIB value of the lumen's blood flow signal before and after stenosis [13]. These indices could improve the diagnostic capability of IVUS for ischemia, suggesting that functional assessment can be added without using FFR at the time of PCI, which may contribute to improved clinical outcomes. Lee et al. developed a machine learning algorithm for IVUS findings representing FFR ≤0.80 and reported that the algorithm showed good diagnostic performance [14]. In the future, we hope that artificial intelligence will be introduced into IVUS software and that it will be able to perform various functions, such as not only ischemia determination but also treatment strategy suggestion and treatment effect determination.

Advice

There are limitations to ischemia assessment by IVUS, and the MLA and plaque volume of the lesion alone should not be used to determine the indication for PCI. IVUS and FFR are complementary and should be considered in determining the optimal procedure.

References

1. Neumann FJ, Sousa-Uva M, Ahlsson A, et al. 2018 ESC/EACTS Guidelines on myocardial revascularization. Eur Heart J. 2019;40:87–165.
2. D'Ascenzo F, Barbero U, Cerrato E, et al. Accuracy of intravascular ultrasound and optical coherence tomography in identifying functionally significant coronary stenosis according to vessel diameter: a meta-analysis of 2,581 patients and 2807 lesions. Am Heart J. 2015;169:663–73.
3. Waksman R, Legutko J, Singh J, et al. FIRST: fractional flow reserve and intravascular ultrasound relationship study. J Am Coll Cardiol. 2013;61:917–23.
4. Cho YK, Nam CW, Han JK, et al. Usefulness of combined intravascular ultrasound parameters to predict functional significance of coronary artery stenosis and determinants of mismatch. EuroIntervention. 2015;11:163–70.
5. Takagi A, Tsurumi Y, Ishii Y, et al. Clinical potential of intravascular ultrasound for physiological assessment of coronary stenosis: relationship. Circulation. 1999;100:256–61.

6. Park SJ, Kang SJ, Ahn JM, et al. Visual-functional mismatch between coronary angiography and fractional flow reserve. JACC Cardiovascular Interv. 2012;5:1029–36.
7. Jasti V, Ivan E, Yalamanchili V, et al. Correlations between fractional flow reserve and intravascular ultrasound in patients with an ambiguous left. Circulation. 2004;110:2831–6.
8. de la Torre Hernandez JM, Hernández Hernandez F, Alfonso F, et al. Prospective application of pre-defined intravascular ultrasound criteria for assessment of intermediate left main coronary artery lesions results from the multicenter LITRO study. J Am Coll Cardiol. 2011;58:351–8.
9. Kuramitsu S, Matsuo H, Shinozaki T, et al. Two-year outcomes after deferral of revascularization based on fractional flow reserve: the J-CONFIRM registry. Circ Cardiovasc Interv. 2020;13:e008355.
10. Park SJ, Ahn JM, Kang SJ, et al. Intravascular ultrasound-derived minimal lumen area criteria for functionally significant left main coronary artery stenosis. JACC Cardiovasc Interv. 2014;7:868–74.
11. Johnson TW, Räber L, di Mario C, et al. Clinical use of intracoronary imaging. Part 2: acute coronary syndromes, ambiguous coronary angiography findings Part 2: acute coronary syndromes, ambiguous coronary angiography findings, and guiding interventional decision-making: an expert consensus document of the European Association of Percutaneous Cardiovascular Interventions. Eur Heart J. 2019;40:2566–84.
12. Seike F, Uetani T, Nishimura K, et al. Intravascular ultrasound-derived virtual fractional flow reserve for the assessment of myocardial ischemia. Circ J. 2018;82:815–23.
13. Takami H, Sonoda S, Muraoka Y, et al. Comparison between minimum lumen cross-sectional area and intraluminal ultrasonic intensity analysis using integrated backscatter intravascular ultrasound for prediction of functionally significant coronary artery stenosis. Heart Vessels. 2019;34:208–17.
14. Lee JG, Ko J, Hae H, et al. Intravascular ultrasound-based machine learning for predicting fractional flow reserve in intermediate coronary artery lesions. Atherosclerosis. 2020;292:171–7.

How to Predict and Prevent Coronary Artery Rupture?

Satoru Sumitsuji

Point for Comprehensive Utilization
- Understanding the mechanism of coronary artery rupture.
- IVUS information can prevent coronary artery rupture.
- Draw a prediction circle to predict the extensibility of the adventitia.

1 Perforation and Rupture

Coronary artery perforation or rupture is one of the most serious complications of PCI, especially coronary artery rupture, which can cause cardiac tamponade in a short time and death if it is delayed. On the other hand, coronary artery perforation rarely leads to cardiac tamponade in a short time.

The original meaning of the word "perforation" is the penetration of a thin object, and in PCI it refers to the perforation caused by a guidewire. "Rupture" is a larger tear in the material, and in PCI it is a "rupture" of the coronary artery wall due to balloon or stent overdilation.

Many people use the terms "perforation" for coronary artery rupture because the Ellis paper [1], the most famous classic paper on coronary artery perforation and rupture, reported perforation including rupture cases. However, we would like you to distinguish perforation from rupture because they are very different in terms of the above process, the mechanism described later, and prediction by IVUS.

S. Sumitsuji (✉)
Endowed Department of International Cardiology, Osaka University Graduate School of Medicine, Suita, Japan
e-mail: satoru@sumi2g.sakura.ne.jp

J. Honye (ed.), *Basics of Comprehensive IVUS-Guided PCI*,
https://doi.org/10.1007/978-981-19-5658-4_8

2 Mechanism and Relevant IVUS images of Coronary Artery Rupture

The structure of coronary arteries is composed of intima (including plaque), media, and adventitia. Among these three layers, adventitia has the highest extensibility. The adventitia is composed of collagen fibers and elastic fibers, and the rearrangement of these fibers results in high extensibility even at relatively low pressures [2].

However, no matter how high the extensibility of the adventitia is, there is a limit to its extensibility, and hyperextension can lead to rupture. This is the mechanism of coronary artery rupture. According to a paper by Chen et al. [2], coronary artery adventitia of normal pigs is stretched 1.8 times at 148 $mmHg^2$, which means that a 3-mm vessel can be stretched to 5.4 mm without tearing.

However, based on our experience, it is unlikely that a balloon and/or a stent 1.8 times the diameter of the vessel for the target segment would be used on angiography and/or IVUS. However, coronary artery rupture does occur in reality. The reason for this seems to be "partial hyperextension of the adventitia".

During the bare-metal stent (BMS) era, there was a theory that bigger is better, and we had experienced cases of coronary artery rupture. The images of IVUS at ruptured segment are shown in Fig. 1.

As IVUS images in Fig. 1, "eccentric calcified or fibrous plque with almost no plque area on the opposite side" were present. If only a plaque-free segment on the contralateral side of the eccentric lesion is hyperextended by balloon or stent, even a balloon or stent of the usual size may cause a tear due to hyperextension of adventitia. Actually, in most cases, when balloon was dilated in such eccentric lesion, the boundary between media and adventitia rather becomes dissected due to the difference in the extensibility of media and adventitia. After medial dissection occurs, a longer part of the adventitia will be extended, extensibility decreases, and tears due to hyperextension do not occur. Furthermore, if calcified lesion was modified by

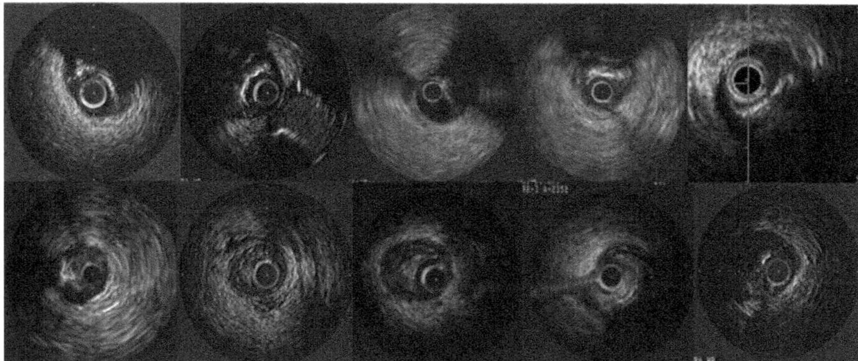

Fig. 1 Preoperative IVUS images at the site of coronary artery rupture after stenting. The upper panel shows eccentric calcified lesions and the lower panel shows eccentric fibrotic lesions with almost no plaque area on the opposite side

ablation devices, the rate of extension of adventitia is reduced, and rupture due to overextension does not occur (Fig. 2).

Figure 3 shows the IVUS findings of different extension status of adventitita in different situation. Upper: adventitia hyperextension without medial dissection. Middle: less extension after medial dissection created. Bottom: less adventitita extension after calcified lesion modification.

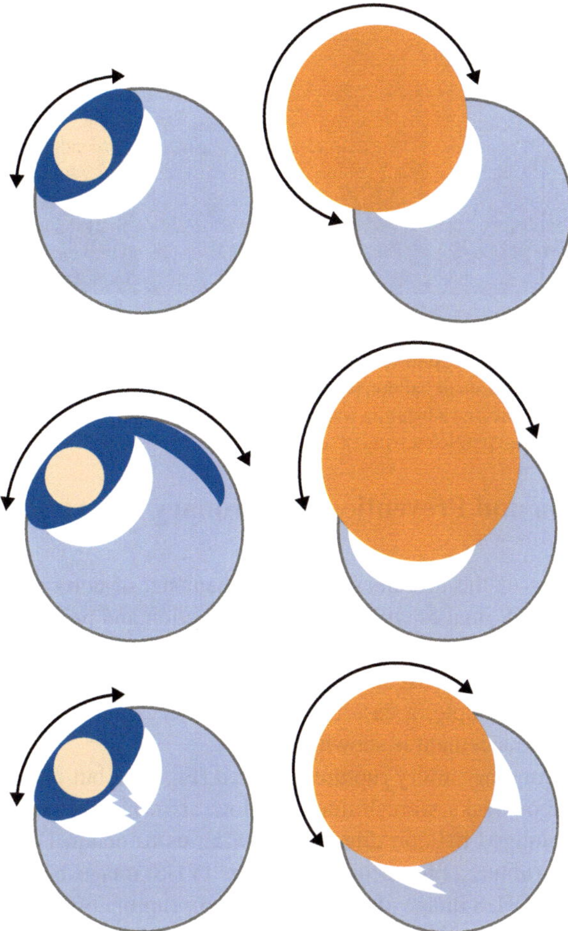

Fig. 2 How to prevent overstretch and rupture of the adventitia. The upper panel shows a situation in which the contralateral side of an eccentric lesion is overstretched. When the adventitia is overstretched beyond its extension limit, a break, or coronary artery rupture, occurs. The middle panel shows a situation in which the rate of extension of the adventitia is reduced due to dissection of the tunica media caused by pre-dilation, making it difficult for adventitial overstretch and rupture to occur. The lower panel shows that when the calcified lesion is cracked by a rotablator, subsequent balloon and stent dilation do not cause overstretch of the adventitia. In other words, it is difficult to cause a rupture of the adventitia

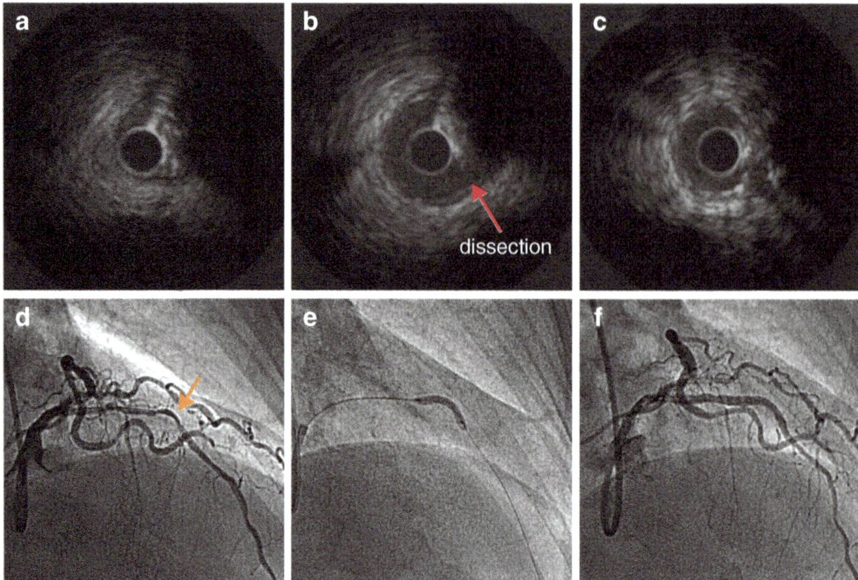

Fig. 3 Typical case of stenting for high rupture risk lesion after medial dissection. Pre- IVUS (**a**) shows an eccentric calcified lesion with a high risk of coronary artery rupture in mid LAD (**d**). After pre-dilatation with a small balloon (**e**), IVUS (**b**) shows a medial dissection at the edge of the calcified lesion. Therefore, the adventitia was not overstretched during subsequent stent (**c**) implantation, and stenting was completed without any trouble (**f**)

3 Prediction and Prevention of Coronary Artery Rupture

An understanding of the aforementioned mechanisms of coronary artery rupture and associated IVUS images will enable the prediction and prevention of coronary artery rupture. An important point is "prediction of hyperextension of the adventitia," and for this purpose, I use the technique of "drawing a virtual circle of dilatation. As a typical example, a case of coronary artery rupture caused by balloon dilation after stent placement is shown in Fig. 4.

In this case, coronary artery rupture occurred (Fig. 4a), but fortunately, contrast medium and blood leaks were limited (yellow arrowhead) and hemostasis was achieved by prolonged balloon dilation, allowing us to obtain IVUS images after coronary artery rupture. Figure 4b shows the IVUS image before stenting and Fig. 4c shows the IVUS image after coronary artery rupture by post-dilation by balloon after stenting. In the IVUS image in Fig. 4c, the lumen is significantly enlarged, and a hypoechoic area in the perivascular tissue (red arrowhead) that was not seen before treatment (Fig. 4b) can be seen. This newly appeared hypoechoic area is a hematoma image created by hemorrhage from the coronary artery.

Here we draw a virtual balloon circle on the IVUS image. Since the balloon used in the case was 4.5mm non-compliant balloon, a circle with a diameter of 4.5mm was drawn, which was almost the same as the lumen diameter when the coronary artery was ruptured (Fig. 5b).

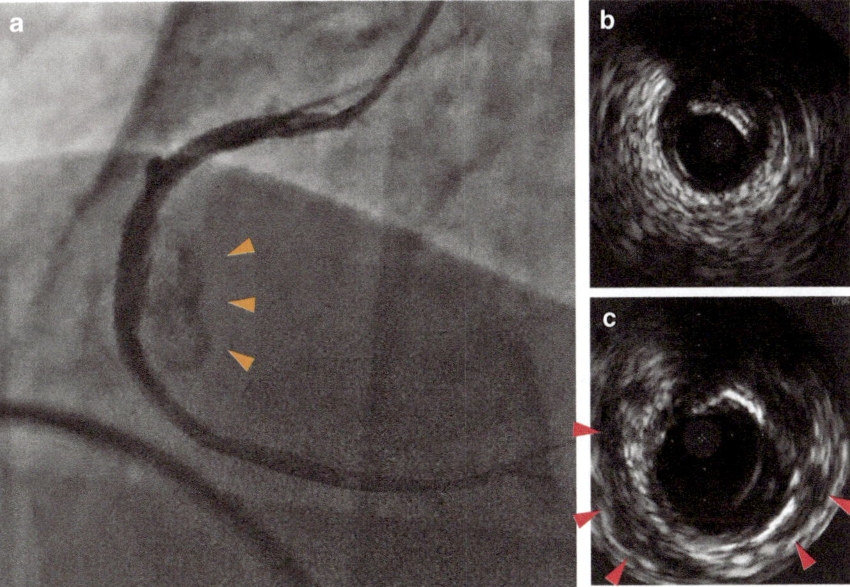

Fig. 4 Coronary artery rupture caused by balloon dilation following drug-eluting stent (DES) implantation. (**a**) A coronary rupture happened by post-balloon dilatation (4.5 mm) after DES implantation. Hemorrhage was limited in the perivascular tissue (yellow arrowhead) and hemostasis was achieved by prolonged balloon inflation. (**b**) Pre-IVUS showed eccentric calcified plaque with plaque-free area on the opposite side of the plqque. (**c**) The post-hemostasis IVUS image reveals a continuous hypoechoic region (4 o'clock) from the lumen to the peri-coronary tissue, indicating that this is the site of coronary rupture

Furthermore, let us apply this "virtual circle of balloon" to the IVUS image before PCI (Fig. 5a). You can understand that there is the possibility of "hyperextension of the adventitia"s shown in Fig. 2 and the risk of coronary artery rupture due to hyperextension of the adventitia.

The measured virtual adventitial extension, in this case, was 195%, which is exceeded the extension rate of 180% shown in experiments with porcine adventitia data. Figure 5c shows the situation of adventitial extension with the same size balloon dilation with concentric plaque. The predicted adventitial extension rate is 120%, and coronary artery rupture will not expected to occur.

Here's the Trick

I hope you understand the importance of "drawing a virtual circle" for predicting adventitial extension, and I urge you to perform this procedure when you actually think you have a risk for coronary artery rupture. If IVUS is used correctly, lots of coronary artery ruptures can be avoided.

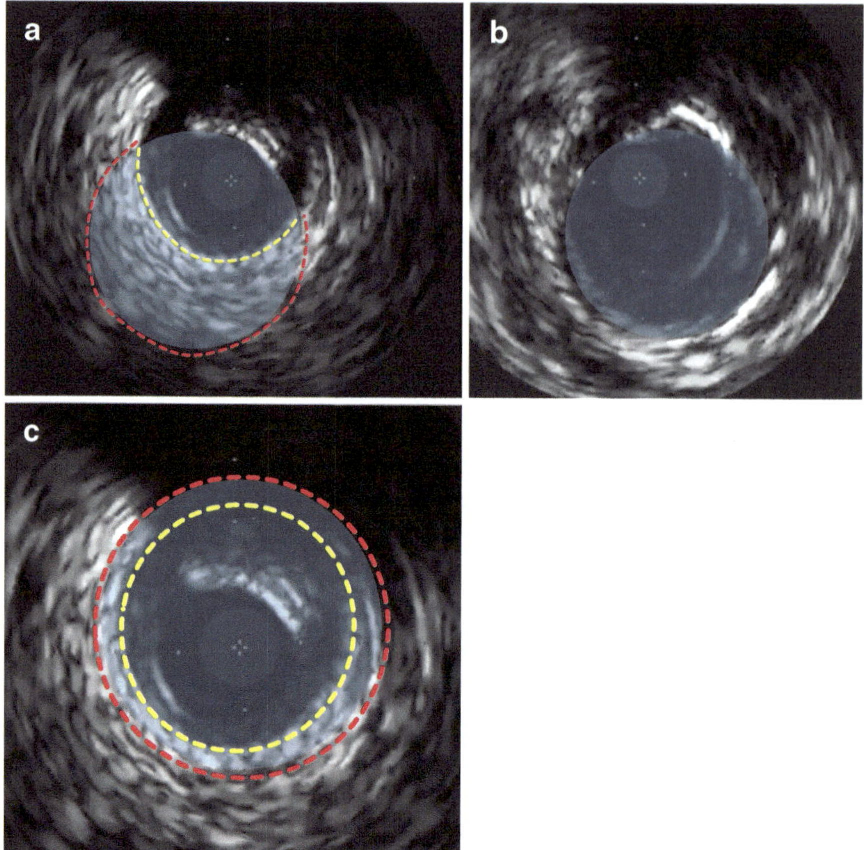

Fig. 5 Example of a virtual expansion circle. (**b**) shows the IVUS image after the coronary rupture with a virtual dilated circle of 4.5 mm in diameter, which is the diameter of the non-compliant balloon that was finally used. It can be seen that the lumen, which was significantly dilated after rupturing of the adventitia, almost coincides with the 4.5-mm virtual dilated circle. (**a**) shows the "state of adventitial stretch" when a non-compliant balloon is assumed to have extended outward from the calcified area and only stretched the adventitia on the opposite side of the eccentric lesion. The length of the red dashed line is almost twice the length of the yellow dashed line, and it is thought that stretch to this extent exceeds the adventitial extension limit and results in the coronary rupture. (**c**) The same virtual circle with a diameter of 4.5 mm was drawn from the center of the coronary artery in pre-PCI IVUS, and the "state of an adventitial stretch" was considered when the entire adventitia was stretched uniformly. When the whole adventitia is stretched, the rate of adventitial extension is about 1.2 times, and rupture due to overstretching does not occur, which means that coronary rupture does not occur

4 Summary

We all know that coronary artery rupture is a lethal complication. As described in this section, I would like you to understand that IVUS can predict coronary artery rupture, and I would like you to perform PCI keeping in mind that coronary artery rupture will not occur as long as IVUS is used. The key to this is the "virtual circle."

References

1. Ellis SG, Ajluni S, Arnold AZ, et al. Increased coronary perforation in the new device era: incidence, classification, management, and outcome. Circulation. 1994;90:2725–30.
2. Chen H, Liu Y, Slipchenko MN, et al. The layered structure of coronary adventitia under mechanical load. Biophys J. 2011;101:2555–62.

Coronary Artery Dissection, Hematoma, and Bail Out Method

Shinjo Sonoda

For Comprehensive Utilization

- Coronary artery dissection and hematoma are common findings during PCI and should not be overlooked because they can cause acute coronary occlusion. They are seen in a variety of situations, including those caused by guiding catheter manipulation or balloon dilation, those occurring at both edges after stenting (due to abundant residual plaque, calcified plaque, uneven strength of the vessel wall with eccentricity, etc.), and special cases that occur spontaneously.
- When new stenosis appears during PCI or when angiographic haziness occurs, IVUS is useful to determine the cause of the stenosis (coronary spasm, dissection, hematoma, or peripheral embolization).
- Because dissection and hematoma can be fatal, appropriate bailout should be performed with careful reading of angiograms and IVUS.

Supplementary Information The online version contains supplementary material available at https://doi.org/10.1007/978-981-19-5658-4_9.

S. Sonoda (✉)
Department of Cardiovascular Medicine, Faculty of Medicine, Saga University, Saga, Japan
e-mail: ssonoda@cc.saga-u.ac.jp

J. Honye (ed.), *Basics of Comprehensive IVUS-Guided PCI*,
https://doi.org/10.1007/978-981-19-5658-4_9

1 What Is Coronary Dissection?

A phenomenon in which the coronary arterial wall separates between the intima and media, detaching from the vessel wall and forming a flap. It tends to occur between fibrous plaque and calcified plaque.

A superficial dissection (intimal dissection), in which the dissection occurs only in the intima, is described as a tear. A medial dissection, in which the dissection extends to the media, is called a dissection (Figs. 1 and 2).

The causes of dissection are listed in Table 1. From the angiographic findings, they are classified as shown in Table 2.

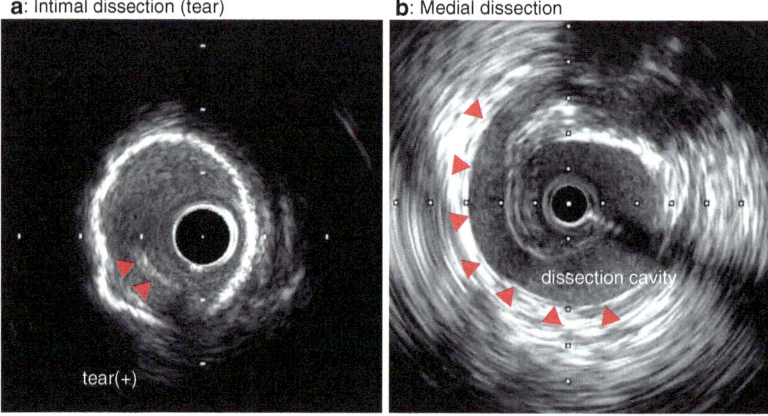

Fig. 1 IVUS image of coronary artery dissection (Video S1: video). (**a**) Intimal dissection (tear). (**b**) Medial dissection

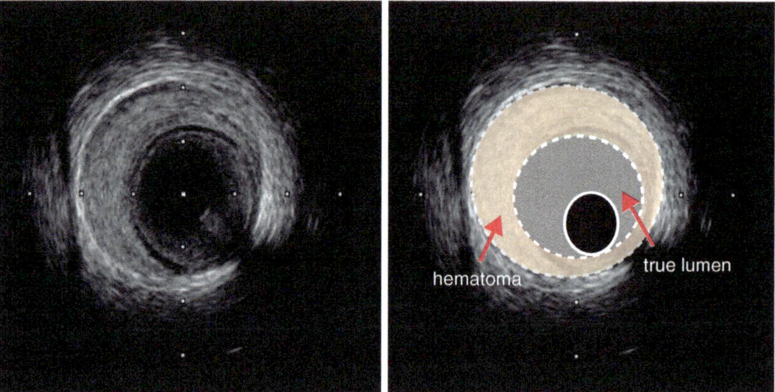

Fig. 2 IVUS image of hematoma. Intramural hematoma: Blood accumulation in the media, crescent- or helmet-shaped, with inward thrust of the internal elastic membrane and outward thrust of the external elastic membrane. A uniform, high-intensity (white), granular echogenicity image is present, reflecting the presence of congestive blood. Fibrin clots within a hematoma that have been present for a period of time present as a hypo (black) echo. A saline or contrast staining also produces a hypo (black) echoic image. Hematoma, true lumen

Table 1 Causes of coronary artery dissection

1. Due to ostial injury by guiding catheter
2. Associated with guidewire manipulation
   Complex lesions with flaps or ulcers, tortuous lesions, chronic total occlusion, bifurcation stenting (guidewire straying into the side branch, formation of a dissection cavity by guidewire)
3. Associated with balloon dilatation or stent implantation occurs at the edge of the stent or within a side branch
4. Spontaneously
   Spontaneous coronary artery dissection (SCAD), etc.

Table 2 NHLBI classification

Type A	Small radiolucent areas within the lumen
Type B	Parallel tract or a double lumen, with no persistence of contrast media
Type C	Contrast media is outside the lumen with pooling of contrast after the lumen has been cleared
Type D	A spiral defect of contrast media
Type E	Dissection with persistent filling defect in the lumen
Type F	Dissection with total occlusion of the lumen and no distal antegrade flow

Attention here
Type C to type F is considered to be at high risk of acute coronary occlusion and require urgent treatment
*NHLBI: National Heart, Lung, and Blood Institute

2 What Is a Hematoma?

If reentry is not created in a dissection that extends to the media, the distal end where the dissection occurs becomes a blind end, causing blood (and contrast medium with saline, etc.) accumulation in the dissection cavity and formation of a hematoma. It is more likely to occur in the eccentric and less plaque areas.

There are two types of hematoma: intramural hematoma and extramural hematoma (Fig. 2). The former is broadly classified as a "dissection."

It is not uncommon to see a combination of dissection and hematoma. If the dissection is visible on coronary angiography, it is more likely to be a dissection extending into the media on IVUS, and if it appears hazy, it is more likely to be a tear in the intima on IVUS. An intramural hematoma is a hematoma within the adventitia, which often drains the true lumen and causes myocardial ischemia, requiring immediate treatment. On the other hand, extramural hematoma is a phenomenon associated with coronary artery perforation, and careful attention should be paid to the perforation. In some cases, hemostatic manipulation is necessary.

3 Spontaneous Coronary Artery Dissection (SCAD)

A representative idiopathic coronary artery dissection is a spontaneous coronary artery dissection (SCAD).

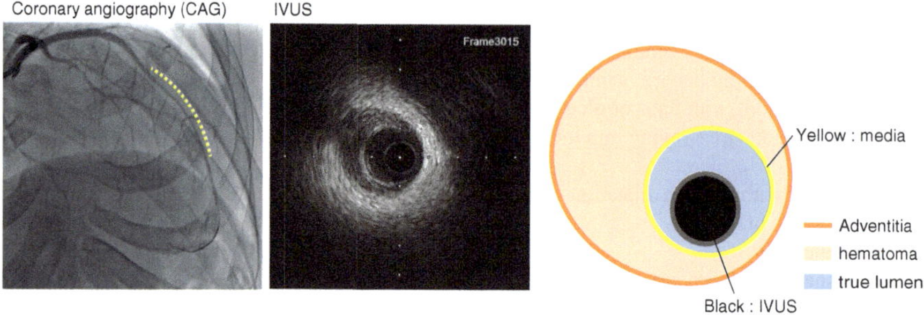

Fig. 3 Case 1: A 42-year-old female, chest pain, close examination. Coronary angiography (CAG), Yellow: media, Black: IVUS, Adventitia, hematoma, true lumen

SCAD is a non-atherosclerotic coronary artery disease. Risk factors include pregnancy, mental and physical stress, and fibromuscular dysplasia, and it is said that nearly 20% will be repeated. Initial diagnosis is important, and IVUS is useful for diagnosis. Figure 3 shows a case of SCAD.

4 What Are the Characteristics of Plaques that May Predict the Development of Dissection and Hematoma?

Dissection rarely occurs in a normal vessel without plaque accumulation (rather, it is a hematoma). Dissection is more likely to occur when the vessel wall has plaque resistant to dilatation, and when there is a combination of plaque volume, uneven wall strength (often adjacent to calcium), and eccentricity (with a relatively normal vessel wall).

5 Situations of Dissection and Hematoma Formation Associated with PCI Procedures

5.1 Ostial Injury by Guiding Catheter

When plaque is present at the entry site, the position of the guiding catheter should be carefully manipulated during coronary angiography and PCI procedures. The position of the guiding catheter should be checked for coaxial engagement. For prevention, it is important to check the pressure waveform if it is wedged, or if the guiding catheter is in deep engage.

In recent years, the use of optical coherence tomography (OCT) for PCI has been increasing. It is important to note that contrast flushing can cause dissection and hematoma formation, which may be a serious situation. Figure 4 shows a representative case.

5.2 *Dissection Associated with Guidewire Manipulation*

Coated wires or relatively stiff wires can easily stray into subintima during PCI for chronic total occlusion or after plain old balloon angioplasty (POBA). The basic principle is to manipulate a guidewire carefully confirming coronary artery track under fluoroscopy.

5.3 *Dissection and Hematoma Associated with Balloon Dilation and Stenting*

Balloon sizing is important in the prevention of malignant dissection formation. The sizing method should be based on a ratio of 0.9 to 1.2 to the reference vessel diameter observed by IVUS.

Smaller sizing is recommended for tortuous or calcified lesions because balloon dilation can easily result in deep dissection. If calcification is severe and poor dilation is anticipated, a scoring balloon, cutting balloon, or rotational atherectomy should be considered.

After stenting, dissection may occur at either stent edge (proximal < distal), resulting in acute occlusion. Stent edge dissection is more likely to cause severe ischemia when it occurs at the distal end than at the proximal end because the flap promotes occlusion.

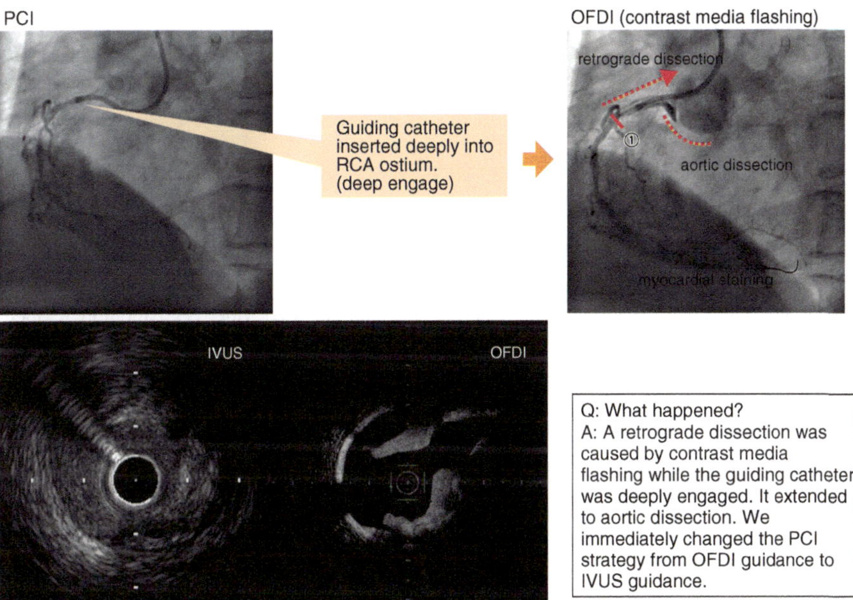

Q: What happened?
A: A retrograde dissection was caused by contrast media flashing while the guiding catheter was deeply engaged. It extended to aortic dissection. We immediately changed the PCI strategy from OFDI guidance to IVUS guidance.

Fig. 4 Case 2: A 67-year-old male, chest pain (BMS restenosis in RCA#1–2)

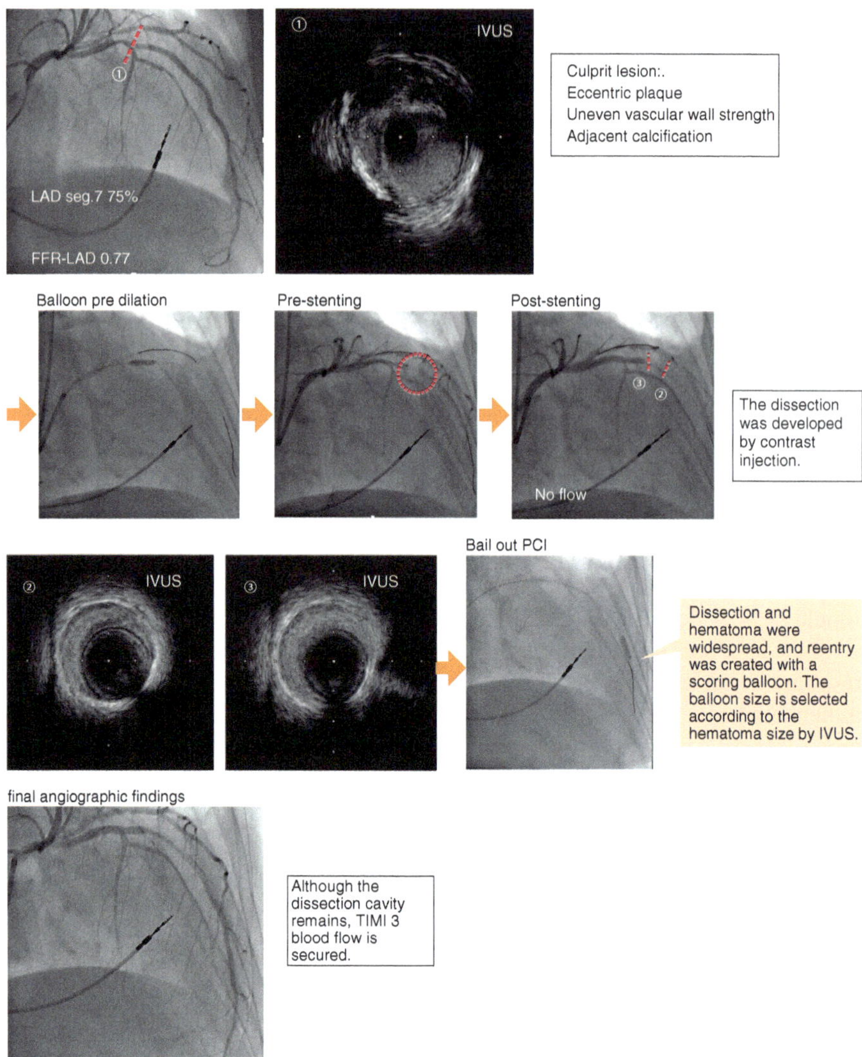

Fig. 5 Case 3: A 71-year-old woman (Video S2: hematoma, video, Video S3: bailout PCI, video)

In general, IVUS can prevent stent edge dissection by selecting a stent/balloon size between the distal reference vessel diameter and the lumen diameter (mid-wall sizing) rather than media-to-media sizing.

Fig. 5 shows an example of a hematoma at the distal end of a stent that was bailed out with a scoring balloon.

5.4 Bail out Method for Coronary Dissection and Hematoma

If there are angiographic haziness in a treated lesion, or if new stenosis develops proximal or distal to the lesion, coronary spasm or dissection/hematoma may have occurred. First, nitrates should be administered. If there is still no improvement, IVUS should be performed to identify the cause. Contrast injection should be avoided to prevent further deterioration of the situation.

When dissection is observed, it is important to evaluate the location and length of the dissection, the extent of the dissection, and whether it affects side branches. As mentioned earlier, it is important to understand that stent edge dissection is more likely to obstruct blood flow in the distal than in the proximal (Fig. 6).

The endpoint of treatment is that the flap does not expand over time and the lumen is well preserved. Intimal dissection or medial dissections less than 60° on IVUS will not cause narrowing of the lumen by the flap (Fig. 7). If there is no luminal narrowing or decreased distal blood flow after 5–10 min, no additional treatment is needed, and most dissections heal well in the chronic phase.

On the other hand, if the dissection is more than 90° or the hematoma is aggravated over time, the entry point should be stented to prevent luminal occlusion. Alternatively, a scoring balloon can create a reentry (IVUS is used to measure the diameter of the vessel at the hematoma site to determine the balloon size). As a result, the true lumen expands due to decompression of the false lumen (Fig. 5).

Advice

The presence or absence of dissection or hematoma after balloon dilatation or stenting should be accurately evaluated not only by angiography but also by IVUS. Once a dissection or hematoma occurs, it is important to determine if it needs to be treated immediately.

IVUS is very useful in accurately determining the location, extent of the dissection or hematoma, and whether it affects the side branches. Furthermore, IVUS provides us with appropriate treatment strategies without contrast media [1, 2].

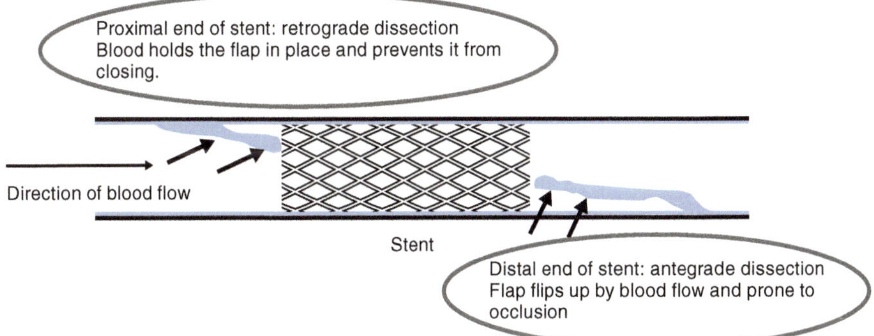

Fig. 6 Key points for prediction of vessel occlusion at stent edge

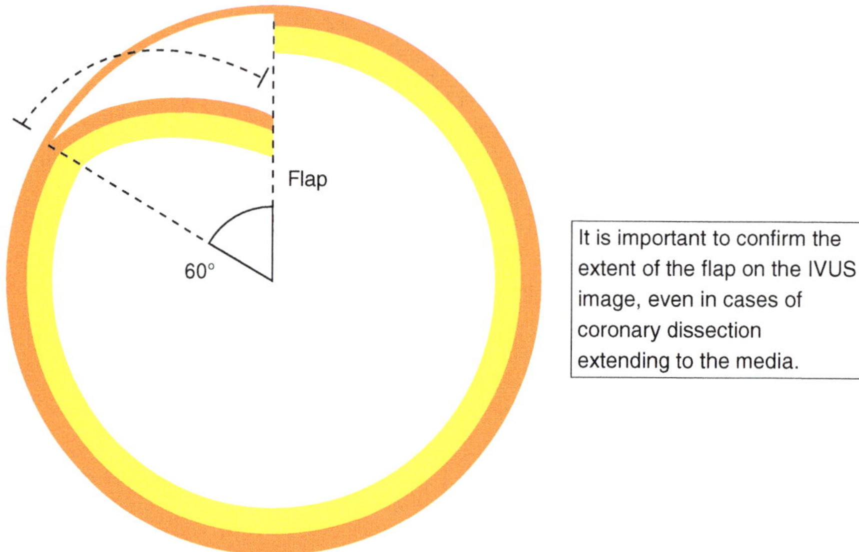

Fig. 7 Flap that can be observed over time

References

1. Saito Y, Sonoda S, Hibi K, et al. Clinical expert consensus document on standards for measurements and assessment of intravascular ultrasound from the Japanese Association of Cardiovascular Intervention and Therapeutics. Cardiovasc Interv Ther. 2020;35:1–12.
2. Sonoda S, Honda Y, Kobayashi Y, et al. Current clinical use of intravascular ultrasound imaging to guide percutaneous coronary interventions. Cardiovasc Interv Ther. 2020;35:30–6.

Mechanisms of Slow Flow/No Reflow Phenomena and How to Deal With

Kenichi Fujii

Points for Comprehensive Use

- Do not focus only on IVUS images.
- The most reliable IVUS finding is the presence of an attenuated plaque.
- Not only a single cross-section but also longitudinal extension is important.

Slow flow and no reflow are often confused in clinical practice, but they are completely different phenomena. No reflow is a reperfusion injury that occurs mainly in patients with acute myocardial infarction, in which myocardial blood flow to the infarcted area fails despite revascularization of the infarcted-related lesion. Since capillaries are structurally destroyed along with myocardial necrosis and capillaries are compressed due to myocardial edema, blood flow from small arteries to capillaries to small veins is blocked. As a result, the blood flow velocity at the epicardial surface of the coronary artery is reduced, resulting in contrast delay in coronary angiography.

Although myocardial contrast echocardiography can be used for diagnosis [1], in the Cath lab it is possible to diagnose systolic flow reversal using a Doppler flow wire [2] or bimodal temperature changes using a pressure wire with a temperature sensor [3]. There are no reports showing that the technique of PCI or plaque characteristics before PCI are related to the occurrence of this phenomenon, and it is almost impossible to predict it by IVUS.

On the other hand, not only in cases of acute myocardial infarction but also in coronary interventions, contrast delay may be observed immediately after balloon dilation or stent implantation for lesions containing unstable plaques or relatively

K. Fujii (✉)
Division of Cardiology, Department of Medicine II, Kansai Medical University, Hirakata, Osaka, Japan
e-mail: fujiik@hirakata.kmu.ac.jp

J. Honye (ed.), *Basics of Comprehensive IVUS-Guided PCI*,
https://doi.org/10.1007/978-981-19-5658-4_10

fresh thrombi. Mechanical stimulation of the plaque causes some lipids and other contents within the plaque to disrupt and fragment, which embolizes the peripheral coronary arteries, increasing coronary resistance and decreasing blood flow velocity. This phenomenon is called "slow flow." Since slow flow is caused by embolization of plaque contents as described above, it can be predicted to some extent by evaluating tissue characteristics of the plaque using IVUS images.

In this section, we describe the slow flow phenomenon, which can be predicted to some extent by IVUS images.

1 In Predicting Slow Flow

As described above, slow flow during PCI is caused by mechanical stimulation of the plaque, which causes some plaque contents to disrupt and fracture, and these contents embolize in the peripheral coronary arteries. Therefore, it is easy to imagine that histological characteristics of the plaque are highly related to slow flow phenomenon. However, when we are asked whether it is only plaque characteristics that are related to slow flow phenomenon, the answer is "no." Of course, the size of a balloon or a stent, dilatation pressure, and size of the vascular bed also contribute to slow flow phenomenon [4].

It is important to note that factors that cause slow flow during PCI are multifactorial, and in clinical practice, it is necessary to predict the occurrence of slow flow based on a combination of factors other than plaque characteristics and the circumstances under which PCI is performed.

2 Predicting Slow Flow from IVUS Images

When asked which plaque has the highest risk of slow flow, many people may think of unstable plaque. It is unlikely that collagen fibers or calcium components detach and cause peripheral embolization, and it is also unlikely that extracellular matrix as seen in pathological intimal thickening or extracellular fat that does not form a lipid core, forms a mass and causes embolization. As for the healed plaque, although it depends on the period of time since thrombus was formed, if it is not in the acute phase after the onset of acute coronary syndrome, the tissue would be organized and become very sparse extracellular matrix, and collagen fibers would proliferate and become hard tissue so that risk for distal embolization would be low. On the other hand, mature atheroma, the so-called unstable plaque, has a large necrotic core inside, and this large necrotic core is considered to have a high risk of disruption and forming a mass as a result of mechanical stimulation by a balloon or a stent, resulting in embolism.

Because these slow flow phenomena occur frequently in acute coronary syndromes, it is often assumed that thrombus formed in the culprit lesion causes embolism, however, a part of necrotic core disrupted from the plaque often causes embolism rather than a thrombotic component [5]. Therefore, how to identify unstable plaque by IVUS is directly related to the prediction of slow flow phenomenon. Based on previous clinical studies and the experience of many IVUS experts, prediction of unstable plaques by IVUS is often based on (1) low echoic plaque, (2) attenuated plaque, and (3) positive remodeling.

3 Low Echoic Plaque

A low echoic plaque is also described as a plaque containing an echolucent area or a lipid pool-like image, but we think that we are basically looking at the same thing. Since Yamagishi et al. [6] reported in 2000 that patients with low echoic plaques have a higher risk of developing acute coronary syndromes in the future, grayscale IVUS has become the standard for diagnosing unstable plaques. In the clinical setting, stenting a lesion with a low echoic plaque may cause slow flow phenomenon (Fig. 1).

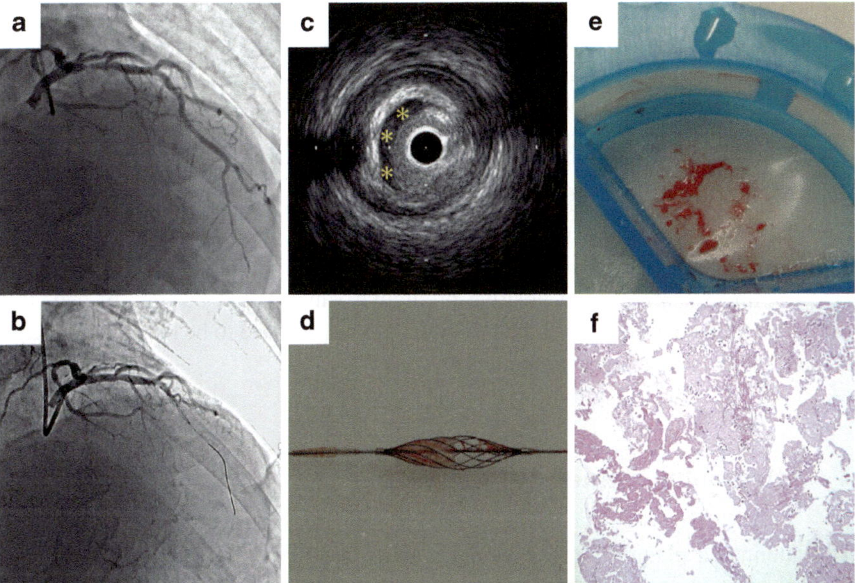

Fig. 1 A case of low echoic plaque with slow flow phenomenon. A highly stenotic lesion in the proximal left anterior descending artery (**a**). When the lesion was observed by IVUS before PCI, a low echoic plaque was observed at 7–12 o'clock (*) (**c**). When the stent was implanted with a distal protection device because of a probable slow flow phenomenon, a filter slow flow phenomenon occurred (**b**). Macroscopic images of the retrieved distal protection device showed that plaque debris was trapped (**d**, **e**). Pathological sections showed necrotic cores with inflammatory cell infiltration (**f**)

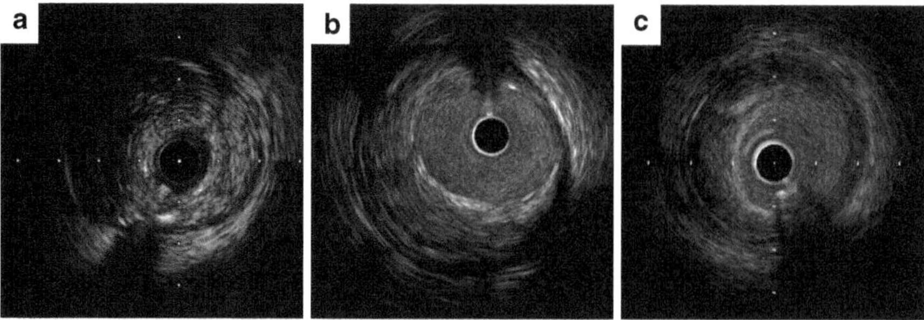

Fig. 2 IVUS image of low echoic plaque. For (**a**), there is a clear low echoic region at 9 o'clock. Both (**b**) and (**c**) have a relatively low echoic region at 7–9 o'clock, but the judgment may differ depending on the observer

It is a fact that low echoic plaque is the most common plaque histology in patients with slow flow phenomenon, however, the positive predictive value is not high. In other words, only a small percentage of low echoic plaques cause slow flow phenomenon, which reduces its clinical significance. Although there are several factors that contribute to the low positive predictive value of low echoic plaques, the two main factors are as follows (i) low diagnostic accuracy of low echoic plaque and (ii) the fact that low echoic plaque is very frequently observed in clinical practice.

The problem with (i) is that the definition of "low echoic" or "low echogenicity" is ambiguous. Figure 2 shows three IVUS images. How can the presence of a low echoic plaque be determined? Fig. 2a shows a typical low echoic plaque, but IVUS images b and c may be judged differently by different observers.

In a previous consensus document on IVUS, plaque characteristics were classified into three categories: fibrous, lipidic, and calcific [7, 8], and this classification is widely used in clinical practice. Therefore, if Fig. 2b, c are classified as low echoic plaques in (ii), a large number of plaques will be diagnosed as low echoic plaques, and sensitivity and positive predictive value would be low. In fact, in a previous ex vivo *study,* 67% of the IVUS images determined to be low echoic plaque actually contained lipid components [9].

4 Attenuated Plaque

The attenuated plaque is most widely used to predict slow flow phenomenon in clinical practice. In the presence of a reflector such as calcium or stent strut (metal), ultrasound signals from the catheter do not penetrate the reflector, and all the signal is backscattered, resulting in an acoustic shadow behind the reflector.

An attenuated plaque is one in which ultrasound signals are attenuated within the plaque and the structure behind the plaque is obscured, despite the absence of calcium or metal (Fig. 3). Because this is a relatively new concept originating in Japan, it has not been clearly described in previous consensus documents [7]. In previous clinical trials, PCI for plaques with attenuated plaques was reported to be an independent contributing factor to the occurrence of slow flow phenomenon [4, 10].

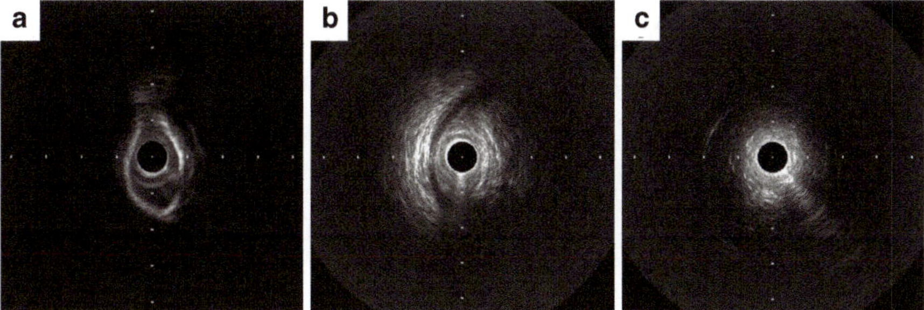

Fig. 3 IVUS image of attenuated plaque. (**a**) Acoustic shadow due to calcification (calcium) within the intima. (**b**) Eccentric attenuated plaque (<180°). (**c**) Circumferential attenuated plaque (360°)

IVUS findings	slow flow (+) event	slow flow (+) total amount	slow flow (–) event	slow flow (–) total amount	odds ratio (95% confidence interval)
Eccentric plaque	31	45	184	415	2.76(1.42-5.40)
Plaque rupture	79	107	227	624	4.51(2.59-7.86)
Attenuated plaque	54	80	93	427	8.30(2.85-24.15)
Low echoic plaque	69	129	251	698	2.65(0.95-7.43)

0.01 0.1 1 10 100
slow flow (+) slow flow (–)

Fig. 4 Relationship between IVUS findings and slow flow phenomenon by meta-analysis. The odds ratio for the occurrence of slow flow phenomenon increased in the order of attenuated plaque, plaque rupture, eccentric plaque, and low echoic plaque

The results of the meta-analysis (Fig. 4) showed that the odds ratio for the occurrence of slow flow was highest for the attenuated plaque, although simple comparison was not possible because of differences among the clinical studies analyzed [10]. However, the odds ratio for the occurrence of slow flow phenomenon was highest for the attenuated plaque [10]. A recent report from Japan also demonstrated that the attenuated plaque was an independent contributing factor for the occurrence of slow flow phenomenon (odds ratio: 3.38, 95% confidence interval: 1.70–6.72) [4].

Attenuated plaque is an unstable plaque, which has been supported by previous ex vivo imaging studies. Yamada et al. [11] examined 36 coronary artery samples obtained from autopsy cases by ex vivo IVUS and compared the obtained IVUS images with pathological images. The results showed that the proportion of necrotic cores in the plaque was significantly higher in the attenuated plaque than in the non-attenuated plaque ($13.0 \pm 19.4\%$ vs. $3.9 \pm 8.0\%$, $p = 0.03$), indicating that the plaque was prone to slow flow phenomenon. In our experience, large necrotic cores, microcalcification, and inflammatory cell infiltration were observed in the area showing strong backward attenuation, as shown in Fig. 5, proving that this is a typical unstable plaque image [12].

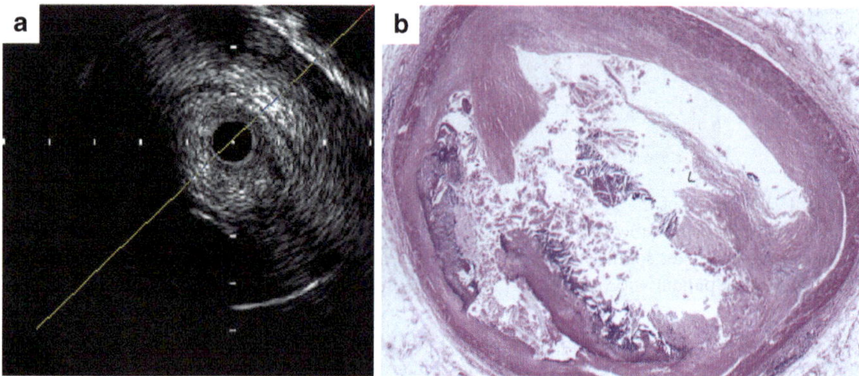

Fig. 5 Pathological images of attenuated plaque. (**a**) Ex vivo IVUS image showing an eccentric plaque with approximately 180°at 5–11 o'clock with posterior attenuation despite the absence of calcium deposition within the plaque. (**b**) Pathological section corresponding to **a**. Large necrotic core with thinning of fibrous cap (fibrous cap tear is an artifact of section preparation)

5 Problems of Attenuated Plaque

As described above, an attenuated plaque can predict a slow flow phenomenon with a higher probability than other IVUS findings, however, we would like to discuss some issues with an attenuated plaque.

One is the definition of an attenuated plaque, which ranges from a relatively narrow angle as shown in Fig. 3b to almost circumferential as shown in Fig. 3c. Although it is supposed that the slow flow phenomenon is related to the size of necrotic core, IVUS images do not provide an accurate measurement of plaque volume because backward attenuation prevents observation of the entire plaque as with calcium. There is a method to measure and define the angle of attenuation, and in cases with concentric plaque, "small angle of attenuation = small necrotic core. However, in cases with eccentric plaque, it does not simply mean "small attenuation angle = small necrotic core."

Because there is no way to solve these problems, it is necessary to predict the size of attenuated plaque based on both proximal and cross-section sections to predict slow flow phenomenon in clinical practice. In the literature, several clinical studies have reported that an attenuated plaque with an angle of 180° or more and an attenuation distance of 5 mm or more in the longitudinal view is more likely to cause slow flow phenomenon [13, 14].

The other issue is that the degree of ultrasound attenuation may be different for different frequencies. Naturally, those images obtained from IVUS of different frequencies are different (Fig. 6), and the angle of attenuation is greater with higher frequencies. Most previous clinical studies used 40 MHz IVUS, but IVUS currently used in clinical practice is mainly 60 MHz. Therefore, it is necessary to re-examine the relationship between attenuated plaque and occurrence of slow flow phenomena with 60 MHz IVUS. If you are using 60 MHz IVUS in clinical practice, you should be aware that you may be overestimating an attenuated plaque a little more than with 40 MHz IVUS.

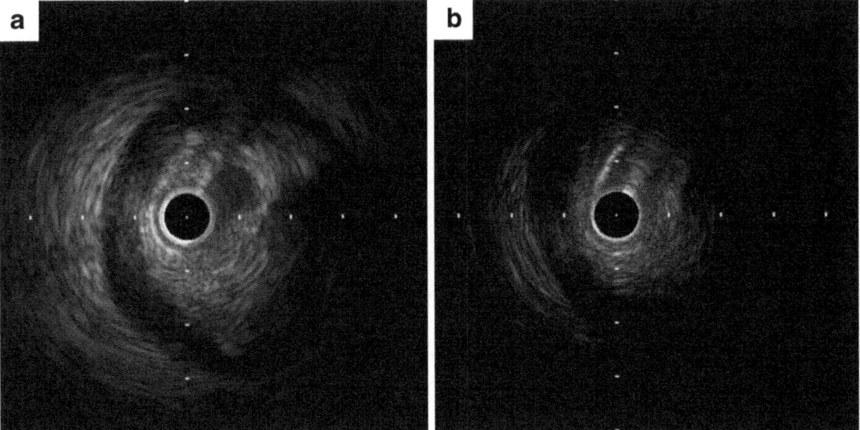

Fig. 6 Evaluation of attenuated plaque by IVUS at different frequencies. The same lesion was observed with 40 MHz IVUS (**a**) and 60 MHz IVUS (**b**), and a comparison between **a** and **b** clearly shows that strong attenuation is found in (**b**)

5.1 *Pay Attention Here*

As mentioned earlier, the greater the frequency, the greater the angle of attenuation is likely to be, so it is necessary to be aware of the frequency of the IVUS being used to diagnose the attenuated plaque.

5.2 *Here's the Trick*

In eccentric attenuated plaques, it is difficult to estimate the size of necrotic core from a circumferential angle. When the device is expanded, the force directly applied to the necrotic core is reduced because mechanical force is initially applied to the healthy side of the plaque (Fig. 7a, b). In the attenuated plaque with a less healthy segment (Fig. 7c), a strong force is applied somewhere in the necrotic core, which increases the risk of disruption or rupture of the fibrous cap and distal embolization of the inner necrotic core. Therefore, when a circumferential attenuated plaque is observed, it is important to understand that slow flow is more likely to occur.

What to do when attenuated plaque is observed and it is determined that it is likely to cause slow flow phenomenon? A prospective, multicenter, randomized trial (VAMPIRE 3) published in Japan demonstrated the efficacy of a distal protection device for treating attenuated plaque [14].

In this study, 200 patients with acute coronary syndrome with attenuated plaques of wider than 180° and longer than 5 mm on IVUS before PCI were randomly assigned to use a distal protection device, and the frequency of slow flow phenomenon during PCI was evaluated. The results demonstrated that the frequency of slow

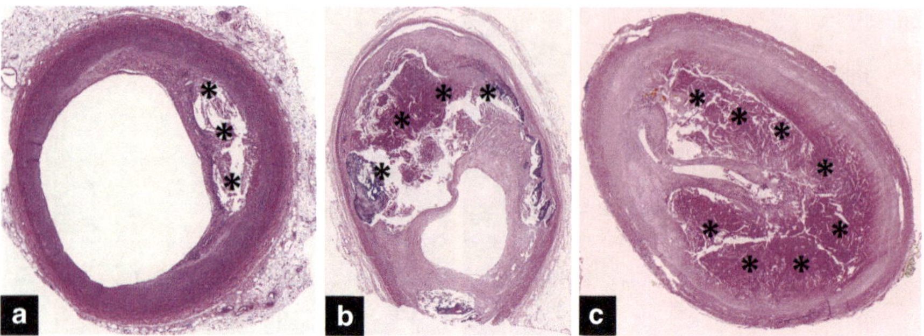

Fig. 7 Size of the necrotic core. Even in plaques classified as fibroatheroma by pathological diagnosis, there are variations in size of the necrotic core (*). (**a**) Small eccentric necrotic core. (**b**) Large eccentric necrotic core. (**c**) Large circumferential necrotic core

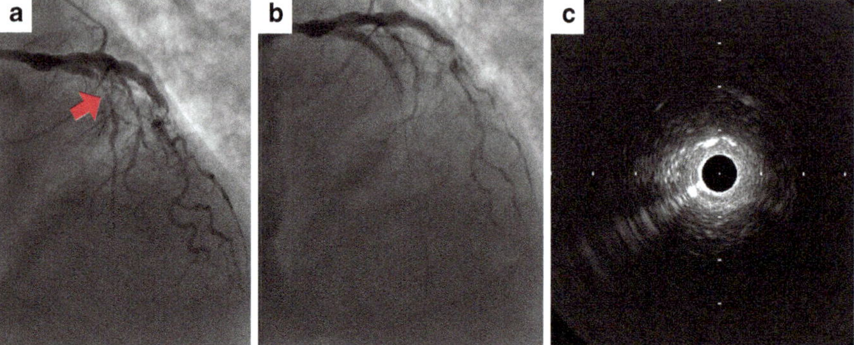

Fig. 8 A case of attenuated plaque with slow flow phenomenon. A case of non-ST-segment elevation acute myocardial infarction. Coronary angiography showed severe stenosis with contrast delay in the middle of left anterior descending artery (→) (**a**), and an attenuated plaque with strong ultrasound signal attenuation in the whole circumference (about 10 mm in the long axis) (**c**) was observed by IVUS before PCI. Immediately after direct stent implantation without a distal protection device, the patient developed slow flow phenomenon with severe chest pain, and ST-segment elevation was developed in anterior leads on electrocardiography (**b**)

flow phenomenon was significantly lower in the group with a distal protection device than in the group without a distal protection device (26.5% vs. 41.7%, $p = 0.026$), providing evidence for usefulness of a distal protection device when performing PCI in patients with attenuated plaques.

We present a case of slow flow experienced by the author (Fig. 8). However, unlike no-reflow phenomenon, slow flow phenomenon that occurs during PCI in patients with acute myocardial infarction is transient, and the degree of myocardial injury is often mild [15]. In addition, operators should know that slow flow phenomenon is often relieved by intracoronary injection of nicorandil or nitroprusside.

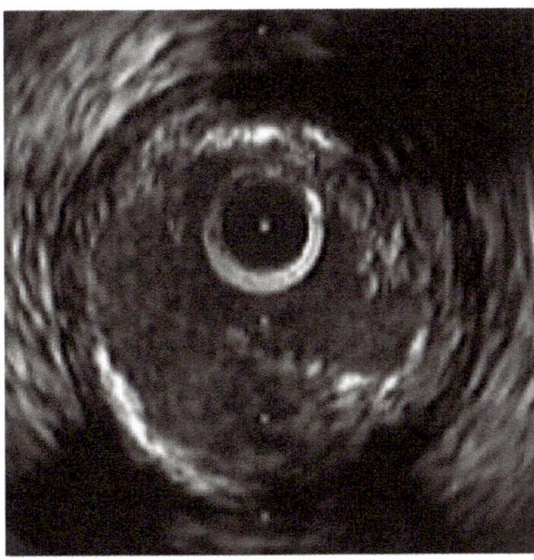

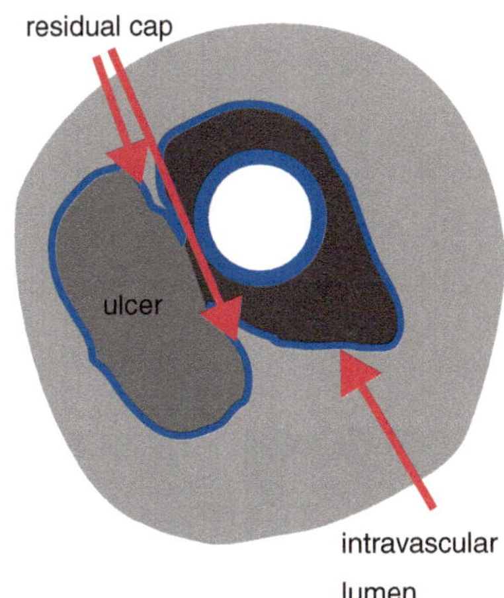

Fig. 9 Plaque rupture image and its schema. On IVUS, the ulcer is often depicted as a cavity connecting to a lumen, and calcium deposits are often seen at the base of the ulcer

6 Plaque Rupture

In the aforementioned meta-analysis, plaque rupture was the IVUS finding with the second highest odds ratio for the occurrence of slow flow phenomenon next to attenuated plaque [10]. Plaque rupture can be seen following disruption of the fibrous cap in unstable plaque and is observed as an ulcer (cavity) connected to the lumen on IVUS (Fig. 9).

Although the mechanism by which plaque rupture causes slow flow phenomenon is obscure, it is probable that residual necrotic core inside the cavity causes distal embolization by mechanical stimulation, or that the lesion with plaque rupture has another unruptured necrotic core nearby. In our previous study, we reported that markers due to myocardial injury were more highly elevated following stent implantation for lesions with plaque rupture than those without [16].

7 Other IVUS Findings

In addition, positive vessel remodeling [17], plaque burden [18], and eccentric plaque [19] have also had been reported to be related to slow flow, however, these are not independent contributors in multivariate analysis [4]. However, these are not independent contributing factors in multivariate analysis [4] so it is difficult to use them clinically to predict slow flow but attenuated plaques and plaque rupture (Fig. 10).

Fig. 10 A case with unstable angina. In patients with unstable angina, coronary angiography shows very tight stenosis with contrast delay in the middle left circumflex, and IVUS images show positive vessel remodeling in which the vessel area at the lesion is larger than reference segments (with attenuated plaque) (**b**) and eccentric plaque (**c**)

References

1. Ito H, Maruyama A, Iwakura K, et al. Clinical implications the 'no reflow' phenomenon: a predictor of complications and left ventricular remodeling in reperfused anterior wall myocardial infarction. Circulation. 1996;93:223–8.
2. Akasaka T, Yoshida K, Kawamoto T, et al. Relation of phasic coronary flow velocity characteristics with TIMI perfusion grade and myocardial recovery after primary percutaneous transluminal coronary angioplasty and rescue stenting. Circulation. 2000;101:2361–7.
3. Fukunaga M, Fujii K, Kawasaki D, et al. Thermodilution-derived coronary blood flow pattern immediately after coronary intervention as a predictor of microcirculatory damage and midterm clinical outcomes in patients with ST-segment-elevation myocardial infarction. Circ Cardiovasc Interv. 2014;7:149–55.
4. Watanabe Y, Sakakura K, Taniguchi Y, et al. Determinants of slow flow following stent implantation in intravascular ultrasound-guided primary percutaneous coronary intervention. Heart Vessel. 2018;33:226–38.
5. Kotani J, Nanto S, Mintz GS, et al. Plaque gruel of atheromatous coronary lesion may contribute to the no-reflow phenomenon in patients with acute. Circulation. 2002;106:1672–7.
6. Yamagishi M, Terashima M, Awano K, et al. Morphology of vulnerable coronary plaque: insights from follow-up of patients examined by intravascular. J Am Coll Cardiol. 2000;35:106–11.
7. Mintz GS, Nissen SE, Anderson WD, et al. American College of Cardiology Clinical Expert Consensus Document on Standards for Acquisition, Measurement and Reporting of Intravascular Ultrasound Studies (IVUS). A report of the American College of Cardiology Task Force on clinical expert consensus documents. J Am Coll Cardiol. 2001;37:1478–92.

8. Saito Y, Kobayashi Y, Fujii K, et al. Clinical expert consensus document on standards for measurements and assessment of intravascular ultrasound from the Japanese Association of Cardiovascular Intervention and Therapeutics. Cardiovasc Interv Ther. 2020;35:1–12.
9. Prati F, Arbustini E, Labellarte A, et al. Intravascular ultrasound insights into plaque composition. Z Kardiol. 2000;89(Suppl 2):117–23.
10. Jang JS, Jin HY, Seo JS, et al. Meta-analysis of plaque composition by intravascular ultrasound and its relation to distal embolization after percutaneous coronary intervention. Am J Cardiol. 2013;111:968–72.
11. Yamada R, Okura H, Kume T, et al. Histological characteristics of plaque with ultrasonic attenuation: a comparison between intravascular. J Cardiol. 2007;50:223–8.
12. Fujii K, Hao H, Shibuya M, et al. Accuracy of OCT, grayscale IVUS, and their combination for the diagnosis of coronary TCFA: an ex vivo validation study. JACC Cardiovasc Imaging. 2015;8:451–60.
13. Endo M, Hibi K, Shimizu T, et al. Impact of ultrasound attenuation and plaque rupture as detected by intravascular ultrasound on the incidence of no-reflow phenomenon after percutaneous coronary intervention in ST-segment elevation myocardial infarction. JACC Cardiovasc Interv. 2010;3:540–9.
14. Hibi K, Kozuma K, Sonoda S, et al. A randomized study of distal filter protection versus conventional treatment during percutaneous coronary intervention in patients with attenuated plaque identified by intravascular ultrasound. JACC Cardiovasc Interv. 2018;11:1545–55.
15. Yamamoto K, Ito H, Iwakura K, et al. Two different coronary blood flow velocity patterns in thrombolysis in myocardial infarction flow grade 2 in acute myocardial infarction: insight into mechanisms of microvascular dysfunction. J Am Coll Cardiol. 2002;40:1755–60.
16. Fujii K, Carlier SG, Mintz GS, et al. Creatine kinase-MB enzyme elevation and long-term clinical events after successful coronary stenting in lesions with ruptured plaque. Am J Cardiol. 2005;95:355–9.
17. Tanaka A, Kawarabayashi T, Nishibori Y, et al. No-reflow phenomenon and lesion morphology in patients with acute myocardial infarction. Circulation. 2002;105:2148–52.
18. Mehran R, Dangas G, Mintz GS, et al. Atherosclerotic plaque burden and CK-MB enzyme elevation after coronary interventions: intravascular ultrasound study of 2256 patients. Circulation. 2000;101:604–10.
19. Iijima R, Shinji H, Ikeda N, et al. Comparison of coronary arterial finding by intravascular ultrasound in patients with "transient no-reflow" versus "reflow" during percutaneous coronary intervention in acute coronary syndrome. Comparison of coronary arterial finding by intravascular ultrasound in patients with "transient no-reflow" versus "reflow" during percutaneous coronary intervention in acute coronary syndrome. Am J Cardiol. 2006;97:29–33.

Predicting Side Branch Occlusion and Techniques for Protecting Side Branches

Kozo Okada and Kiyoshi Hibi

Points for Comprehensive Utilization

- IVUS is useful in predicting side branch occlusions.
- IVUS plays a significant role in guiding treatment of bifurcation lesions.
- Achievements of optimal stent expansion can be evaluated in left main (LMT) bifurcation lesions.

  LMT: Left main coronary trunk.

1 Side Branch Obstruction

In complex PCI for bifurcation or diffuse lesions, side branch occlusion may occur following balloon dilation or stent implantation for the main branch. This is not uncommon, occurring in about 10% of cases. This is a complication that should be avoided as much as possible because if the perfusion area of the side branch is large and a guidewire cannot pass through the side branch, chest pain and ECG abnormalities may occur, and if side branch occlusion persists, it may progress to myocardial infarction.

K. Okada · K. Hibi (✉)
Division of Cardiology, Yokohama City University Medical Center, Minami-ku, Yokohama, Kanagawa, Japan
e-mail: hibikiyo@yokohama-cu.ac.jp

J. Honye (ed.), *Basics of Comprehensive IVUS-Guided PCI*,
https://doi.org/10.1007/978-981-19-5658-4_11

In the multi-center COBIS II registry, 8.4% of 2227 patients with bifurcation lesions had side branch occlusions, and there was a 2.34-fold increase in cardiac death and myocardial infarction in patients with side branch occlusions. In this study, stenosis of 50% or more at the ostium of the side branch on coronary angiography (CAG) was considered as a predictor of side branch occlusion, however, this is not sufficient because 3–6% of patients will have an occlusion even without a ostial stenosis of the side branch. Although it is difficult to prevent side branch occlusion completely, more accurate prediction is important because various measures would be taken if side branch obstruction can be predicted in advance.

IVUS is useful in predicting side branch occlusions and determining strategies for bifurcation lesions because it provides direct visualization of the entire vessel wall and perivascular tissues with sufficient tissue penetration to accurately evaluate morphology of bifurcation lesions.

2 To Predict Side Branch Occlusion on IVUS

The main reasons for side branch occlusion are plaque shift and carina shift.

The authors reported that evaluation of the side branch at the time of IVUS pullback from the main branch is useful for predicting side branch occlusion due to plaque shift [1]. Eighty-one bifurcation lesions with more than 50% stenosis at ostium of the side branch on CAG were evaluated by IVUS pullback from the main branch We classified 81 bifurcation lesions into three groups according to the distribution of plaque: (1) no plaque in the side branch (no side branch lesion group), (2) plaque in the proximal part of the side branch (with side branch lesion group, proximal type), and (3) plaque in the distal part or the entire circumference of the side branch (with side branch lesion group, distal or entire circumference type) (Fig. 1), and evaluated the rate of side branch occlusion.

The rate of side branch occlusion after PCI was significantly higher in the group with side branch lesions (n = 20) than in the group without side branch lesions (n = 61) (35.0% vs. 8.2%, p = 0.003). Furthermore, among patients with side branch lesions, 1 of 14 patients (7.1%) with the proximal type had side branch occlusion, whereas all six patients (100%) with distal or total circumferential type had side branch occlusion. In contrast, plaque shape and distribution in the main branch did not affect the rate of side branch occlusion.

This result suggests that patients with distal or circumferential plaque at ostium of a side branch during IVUS pullback from the main branch are at particularly high risk of side branch occlusion following PCI and side branch protection should be considered. Figure 2 shows a case of side branch occlusion after stenting despite the insertion of a protective wire into the side branch due to the presence of circumferential plaque at ostium of the side branch on IVUS, which was considered to have a high risk of occlusion.

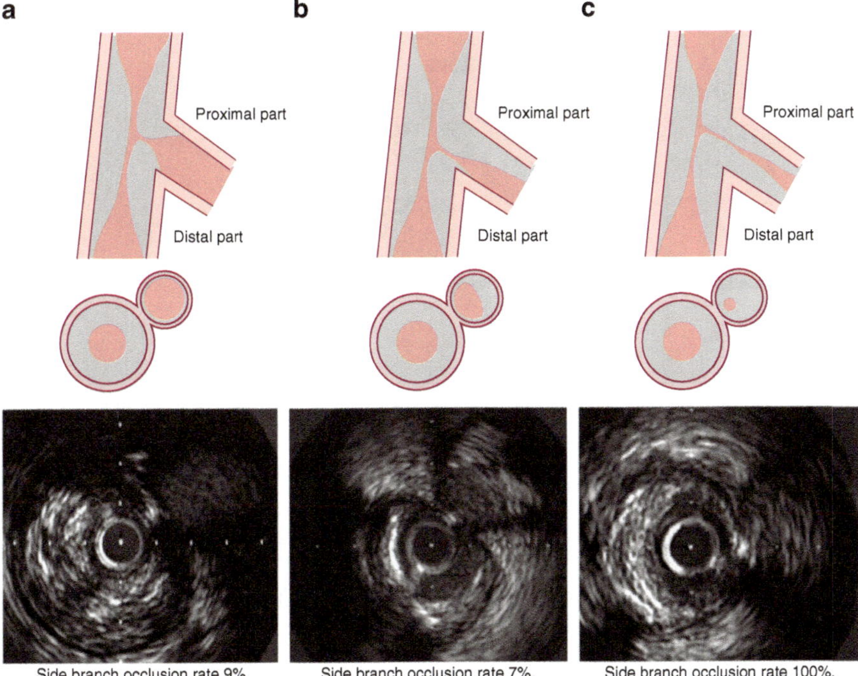

Fig. 1 Classification according to the plaque distribution in the side branches assessed during IVUS pullback from the main branch. Upper row: IVUS classification of bifurcation lesions. (**a**) More than 50% of the lesions are located at the ostium of the side branch on CAG, but no lesions are found in the side branch immediately after the bifurcation (no side branch lesion group). (**b**) Lesions only in the proximal part of the side branches (group with side branch lesions, proximal type). (**c**) Lesions with distal or total circumferential involvement of a side branch (group with side branch involvement, distal or total circumferential type). Lower column: (**a**) IVUS findings in the no side branch lesion group. (**b**) IVUS findings of the proximal type in the group with side branch lesions. (**c**) IVUS findings of the group with side branch lesions of a circumferential type, with little or no lumen within the side branches on IVUS. Proximal part, Distal part, Side branch occlusion rate 9%, Side branch occlusion rate 7%, Side branch occlusion rate 100%

Advice

IVUS is also useful in predicting side branch obstruction due to carina shift. For example, if the bifurcation angle from the main branch to a side branch is shallow and the carina protrudes into the entrance of a side branch on IVUS longitudinal view, the risk of side branch occlusion is high. In addition, if a hard plaque such as calcification exists on the contralateral side of the bifurcation, a stent placed in the main branch may be pushed into the side branch where it has less support, resulting in occlusion of the side branch due to carina shift [2]. In addition, when a large amount of plaque is found in the proximal part of the main branch in bifurcation lesions, a longitudinal plaque shift is more likely to occur at ostium of the side branch.

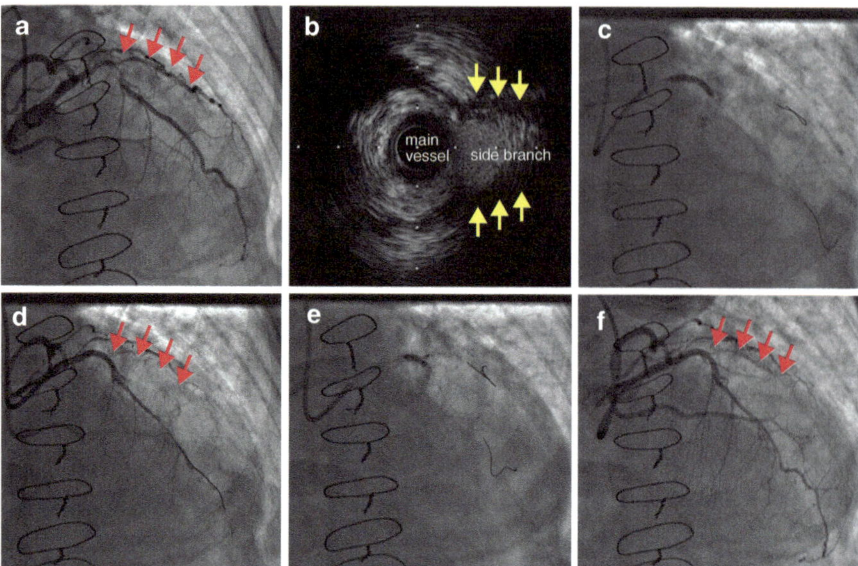

Fig. 2 A case of side branch occlusion. This patient was admitted with a diagnosis of angina pectoris. The CAG showed a 90% stenotic lesion in proximal LAD and a 50% stenosis at ostium of the diagonal branch (**a**). IVUS before PCI demonstrate a circumferential plaque at ostium of the diagonal branch (arrow), which was considered to be at high risk of occlusion (**b**), and an Ultimaster® 2.5 × 15 mm stent was implanted in the LAD after insertion of a protective guidewire into the diagonal branch (**c**). CAG immediately after stent implantation showed that blood flow into the diagonal branch was maintained, but after removal of the protective guidewire, the diagonal branch became occluded (**d**), and the patient complained of chest pain. The guidewire was recrossed from inside of the stent, and a kissing balloon technique was performed to treat the side branch (**e**), which successfully restored blood flow to the lateral side despite dissection at the entry of the side branch (**f**). Main vessel; Side branch

3 Basic Strategies for the Treatment of Bifurcation Lesions

Appropriate evaluation of the lesion and bifurcation-specific techniques are necessary to achieve good outcomes of PCI for bifurcation lesions. IVUS provides accurate information on vessel diameter, degree of stenosis, plaque distribution, presence of calcification, and bifurcation angle of the main branch and side branches, which is useful for predicting side branch occlusion and determining PCI strategy. In addition, IVUS marking technique can be used to accurately correspond the true location of the side branch entry on CAG, which can assist in recrossing the guidewire into the occluded side branch.

On the other hand, when planning a treatment strategy for bifurcation lesions, in addition to IVUS lesion assessment, bifurcation lesion-specific assessments should be considered, including the location of bifurcation lesion, the size of myocardial perfusion area of the target side branch, ease of guidewire recrossing in the event of side branch occlusion, and possibility of overlapping stent struts at the entry of a side branch. In fact, LMT bifurcation lesions often require some side branch technique because they are different from other bifurcation lesions in terms of perfusion area, vessel diameter, bifurcation angle, PCI results, and prognosis. In contrast, for bifurcation lesions other than LMT, balloon dilation or stenting of the side branch should be considered if the perfusion area is large and occlusion rate of the side branch would be high based on CAG or IVUS findings. If the perfusion area is quite small, a strategy with only guidewire protection and no stenting for the side branch should be considered.

Guidewire recrossing for the side branches would be difficult when calcification is present right at bifurcation or when the lesion length in the side branch is long. In addition, overlap stenting in the main branch is often necessary in diffuse long lesions, however, it is not easy to cross a guidewire or balloon through 2-stent struts at the overlapping site of the stent.

4 Side Branch Protection Techniques

The most common technique for side branch protection is guidewire protection, which has been reported to reduce the final rate of side branch occlusion. Two guidewires rather than one guidewire may further reduce the final occlusion rate. This is because removal of one guidewire not only creates space for recrossing a guidewire in case of side branch occlusion, but also makes it easier to recross a guidewire to the occluded side branch because the remaining guidewire serves as a landmark. Even if a guidewire is not able to be recrossed, removal of the second guidewire will increase the space and increase the probability of resuming blood flow to the side branch.

In the aforementioned COBIS II registry, insertion of a protective wire into a side branch did not completely avoid side branch occlusion, however, the final recovery of blood flow in the occluded side branch was greater in patients who had a protective guidewire inserted. It is considered that the space created by removal of the protective guidewire allowed blood flow to be restored, and insertion of two protective wires may further increase the possibility of blood flow restoration as described above.

When the bifurcation angle of the side branch is reversed on CAG or IVUS, it is difficult to select the side branch with conventional guidewire manipulation. Therefore, the reverse wire technique is useful to select the side branch from the distal part using a pre-bent guidewire with a double-lumen catheter. When perfusion area of the side branch is large and large myocardial damage can be predicted in case of side branch occlusion, use of Jailed Balloon Technique or Modified Jailed Balloon Technique [3], or insertion of a penetrating catheter, ASAHI Corsair (manufactured by Asahi Intec) (Jailed Corsair Technique), have also been reported.

5 Bifurcation Lesion Treatment

The key points in the PCI for bifurcation lesions are adequate preparation, stenting for the main branch, and side branch treatment, and IVUS plays an important role in all treatment steps.

5.1 The Role of IVUS in Preparation

For example, adequate preparation before stenting can avoid side branch occlusions and stenoses caused by plaque shift and/or carina shift after stenting. Prior evaluation of plaque distribution and characteristics by IVUS allows appropriate preparation such as balloon dilation including kissing balloon and debulking technique [rotablator or directional coronary atherectomy (DCA)]. Similarly, IVUS information on vessel diameter, lesion length, and residual plaque is useful in determining the optimal stent sizing for stenting.

5.2 The Role of IVUS in the Treatment of Side Branches

In addition, it has been pointed out that the site of guidewire recrossing to the side branch could affect stent expansion following PCI for side branch. If the guidewire can be crossed through the strut as distal as possible to the side branch, distortion of the main stent and incomplete stent apposition are minimized, and good expansion is more likely to be achieved because no struts remain at the ostium of the side branch. In addition to stent expansion and crimping, IVUS can confirm that the guidewire to the side branch crosses through the appropriate distal strut distal at the bifurcation.

5.3 Stent Placement

The basic method is 1-stent strategy.

In PCI for bifurcation lesions, the 1-stent strategy, in which a stent is placed only in the main branch, is simple and has been reported in large-scale clinical trials and meta-analyses to have better outcomes than the 2-stent strategy, in which stents are placed in both main vessel and a side branch [4]. Therefore, balloon dilation for the side branch without thinking should be avoided after stenting the main vessel, but if the side branch becomes severely stenotic or obstructed after stenting, the guidewire should be recrossed to the side branch through the stent strut, and the side branch treatment or stenting should be considered if necessary.

Here's the Trick

Although KBT and proximal optimization technique (POT) are often used during PCI for the side branches, it is important to maintain the proximal part of the main vessel as circular as possible confirming IVUS and to adequately dilate the ostium of the side branches.

5.3.1 When 2-Stent Strategy Is Necessary?

A 2-stent strategy would be necessary if the vessel diameter of the side branch is large (>2.75 mm), if there is a severe stenosis with a large perfusion area, and if the lesion length in the side branch is long (>5 mm), including lesions in the LMT bifurcation.

There are two types of 2-stent technique: stenting the side branch from the beginning (e.g., crush stent, mini-crush stent, and T-and-protrusion (TAP)) and stenting during the procedure (e.g., T-stent and Culotte stent). As with the single-stent strategy, good stent expansion and good apposition of the main vessel and side branches are important for improved outcomes with the 2-stent strategy. In recent years, it has been reported that the use of second-generation and later drug-eluting stents can achieve results equivalent to or better than those of the 1-stent technique [5–7]. Therefore, the 2-stent technique should be recognized as a technique for side branch protection [5–7]. In particular, in LMT bifurcation lesions, it has been reported that the double kissing crush stenting technique was associated with lower rates of revascularization (5.0% vs. 10.3%, $p = 0.029$) and stent thrombosis (0.4% vs. 4.1%, $p = 0.006$) at 3 years compared with provisional stenting.

It has been reported that good stent expansion in LMT bifurcation lesions could improve clinical outcomes. Kang et al. [8] reported that patients with minimum stent area on IVUS that met the optimal expansion criteria (Fig. 3) had

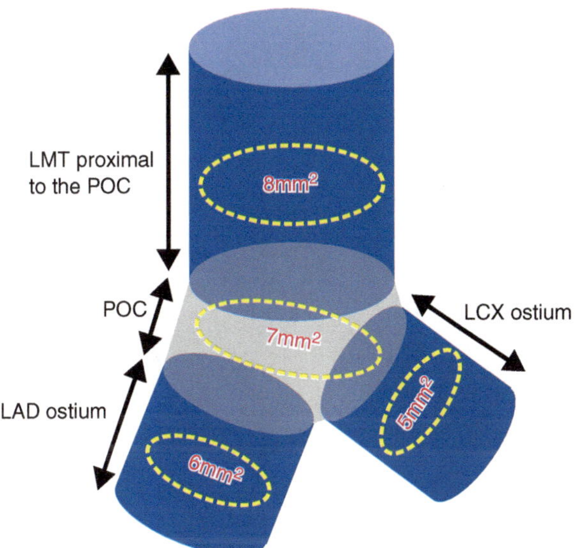

Fig. 3 Optimal stent expansion criteria for the treatment of LMT bifurcation lesions. Kang et al. proposed that optimal stent expansion criteria for the treatment of LMT bifurcation lesions include a minimum stent area of 8 mm^2 at the left main above the polygon of confluence (POC), 7 mm^2 at the POC, 6 mm^2 at ostial LAD (within 5 mm from ostium), and 5 mm^2 at ostial LCX (within 5 mm from ostium). LMT proximal to the POC 8 mm^2; POC 7 mm^2; LAD ostium 6 mm^2; LCX ostium 5 mm^2

significantly lower in-stent restenosis rates at 9 months (5.4% vs. 24.1%, $p < 0.001$) and higher cardiovascular event avoidance rates at 2 years (98 ± 1% vs. 90 ± 3%, $p < 0.001$). The importance of optimal stenting (optimization) by IVUS has been demonstrated.

Fig. 4 shows an example of LMT bifurcation lesion treatment in which good stent expansion was achieved by IVUS.

LCX: Left circumflex artery.
LAD: Left anterior descending artery.

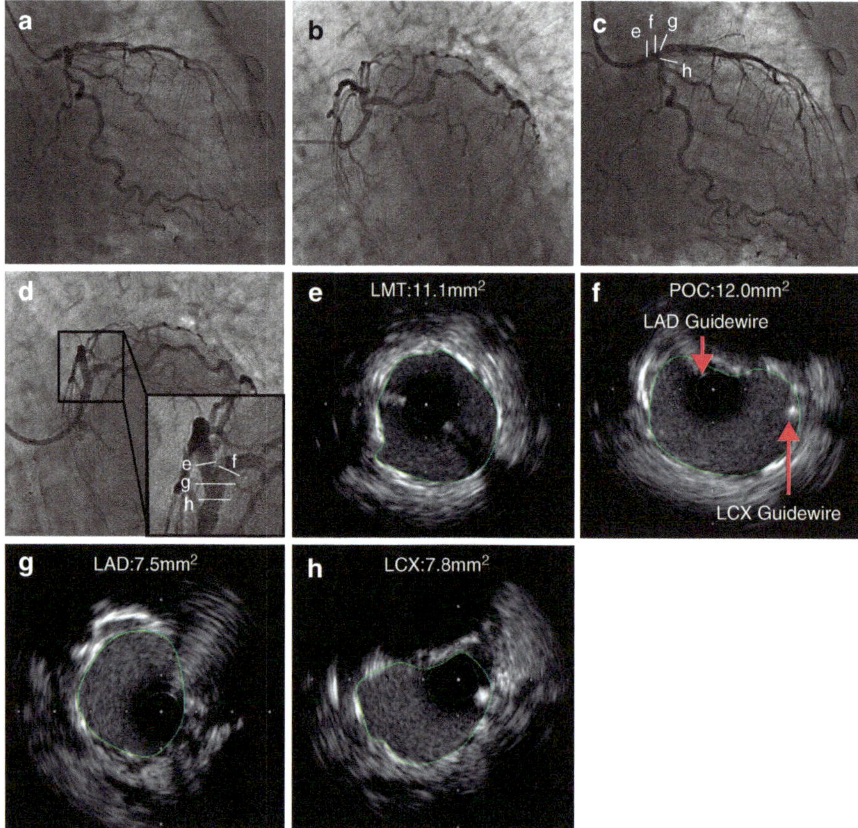

Fig. 4 A representative case of PCI for LMT bifurcation lesion. The patient was admitted with non-ST-segment elevation myocardial infarction, and CAG revealed total occlusion in the mid-RCA and a calcified lesion at LMT bifurcation (90% at the distal LMT, 90% stenosis at the ostial LAD, and 75% stenosis at the ostial LCX)supplying collateral circulation to the lesion in RCA, and a 90% stenosis in the mid-LAD (**a**, **b**). XIENCE Xpedition® 3.0 × 48 mm was implanted in the LAD and SYNERGY™ 3.5 × 16 mm was implanted from the LMT to the LCX using Culotte technique (**c**, **d**). IVUS after stenting confirmed that minimum stent area at the left main (**e**), at the polygon of confluence (POC) (**f**), at the LAD ostium (**g**), and at the LCX ostium (**h**), all met the criteria (Fig. 3) suggested by Kang et al. LMT:11.1 mm^2; POC:12.0 mm^2; LAD Guidewire; LCX Guidewire; LAD:7.5 mm^2; LCX:7.8 mm^2

6 Future Prospects

IVUS is useful not only for predicting side branch occlusions but also for determining PCI strategy and optimal endpoint of bifurcation lesions, which would contribute to improve clinical outcomes. Especially in LMT bifurcation lesions, it is often impossible to achieve PCI without IVUS, and it is important to obtain adequate stent expansion with IVUS.

The OPTIVUS trial is currently underway to evaluate the efficacy of optimal IVUS-guided PCI in patients with severe coronary artery disease (LMT disease and multivessel disease including LAD) using predetermined IVUS criteria for stent expansion (OPTIVUS criteria). This trial will include many bifurcation lesions, including LMTs, and is expected to demonstrate the efficacy of IVUS-guided PCI for these lesions.

References

1. Furukawa E, Hibi K, Kosuge M, et al. Intravascular ultrasound predictors of side branch occlusion in bifurcation lesions after percutaneous coronary. Circ J. 2005;69:325–30.
2. Fujino Y, Attizzani GF, Tahara S, et al. Impact of main-branch calcified plaque on side-branch stenosis in bifurcation stenting: an optical coherence tomography study. Int J Cardiol. 2014;176:1056–60.
3. Tondas AE, Mulawarman R, Trifitriana M, et al. A systematic review of the jailed balloon technique for coronary bifurcation lesion: conventional-jailed balloon technique vs modified-jailed balloon technique. Cardiovasc Revasc Med. 2020; S1533-8389(20)30133-0
4. Ford TJ, McCartney P, Corcoran D, et al. Single- versus 2-stent strategies for coronary bifurcation lesions: a systematic review and meta-analysis of randomized trials with long-term follow-up. J Am Heart Assoc. 2018;7:e008730.
5. Chen X, Li X, Zhang J-J, et al. DKCRUSH-V Investigators: 3-year outcomes of the DKCRUSH-V trial comparing DK crush with provisional stenting for left main bifurcation lesions. JACC Cardiovasc Interv. 2019;12:1927–37.
6. Lee JM, Hahn J-Y, Kang J, et al. Differential prognostic effect between first- and second-generation drug-eluting stents in coronary bifurcation lesions: patient-level analysis of the Korean Bifurcation Pooled Cohorts. JACC Cardiovasc Interv. 2015;8:1318–31.
7. Kumsars I, Holm NR, Niemelä M, et al. Nordic Baltic bifurcation study group: randomised comparison of provisional side branch stenting versus a two- stent strategy for treatment of true coronary bifurcation lesions involving a large side branch: the Nordic-Baltic Bifurcation Study IV. Open Heart. 2020;7:e000947.
8. Kang SJ, Ahn JM, Song H, et al. Comprehensive intravascular ultrasound assessment of stent area and its impact on restenosis and adverse cardiac events in 403 patients with unprotected left main disease. Circ Cardiovasc Interv. 2011;4:562–9.

IVUS Complications and Troubleshooting

Junko Honye

Points for Comprehensive Utilization

- Flushing an IVUS catheter in a coronary artery can cause air emboli.
- If you feel any resistance when removing the IVUS catheter, do not pull it out any further.
- Troubleshooting methods need to be shared with staff in the Cath lab.

IVUS catheter insertion itself has few complications, and coronary spasm which improves with nitric acid administration, was reported to occur in 2.9% of patients [1]. Although there have been rare reports of acute coronary occlusion [2] and thrombotic complications [3]· IVUS catheters have become smaller in diameter and IVUS is safer than when it was first reported. However, it is important to understand probable complications and bailout procedures and to be prepared for just in case.

J. Honye (✉)
Kikuna Memorial Hospital, Yokohama, Kanagawa, Japan
e-mail: jhonye@kmh.or.jp

J. Honye (ed.), *Basics of Comprehensive IVUS-Guided PCI*,
https://doi.org/10.1007/978-981-19-5658-4_12

1 Complications Associated with Routine Procedures

1.1 Appearance of Ischemia

When an IVUS catheter is inserted into a high-grade stenosis before PCI, chest pain and ST-segment elevation on the monitoring system may occur if the observation time is prolonged. Although this is unavoidable for treatment, it is necessary that not everyone concentrate on IVUS images during observation, but someone should take the role of observing ECG and blood pressure monitoring. In any case, ischemia usually resolves quickly after removal of the IVUS catheter, but care should be taken to avoid hemodynamic compromise in severe multivessel disease.

If an AltaView® catheter is used with Terumo's VISICUBE® system, the pullback speed can be set up to 9 mm/sec, and the pullback speed should be changed according to the case.

1.2 Coronary Spasm

Intracoronary nitrates are usually administered prior to insertion of the IVUS catheter, and then IVUS observation is performed. Even so, coronary spasm associated with catheter insertion may occur, but it is quickly relieved by intracoronary administration of nitrates again.

1.3 Dissection

When using an IVUS catheter with a long monorail system (Eagle Eye® or Navifocus® WR), if the IVUS tip is trapped in a lesion or calcification during pullback, the guiding catheter may be pulled in, resulting in dissection at the ostium of the coronary artery. Use of a sheath-type IVUS catheter is recommended for routine PCI.

1.4 Air Embolism

Inadequate air evacuation around the transducer during preparation of the IVUS catheter may result in dark and blurred images during observation (Fig. 1). If several flushes are performed in the coronary artery at this time, air embolization may occur, causing chest pain and ST-segment elevation due to transient slow flow. In addition to proper setup, it is necessary to perform flushing while rotating the imaging core outside the body to remove air bubbles before inserting the IVUS catheter.

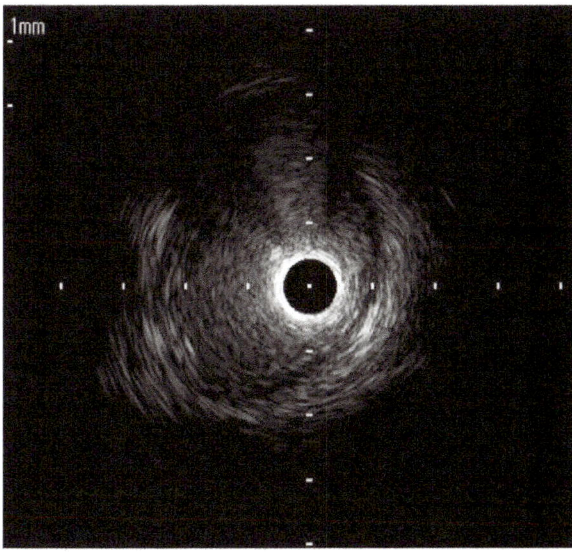

Fig. 1 Air bubbles. If air bubbles around the transducer are insufficiently removed, the image quality is significantly impaired. At this time, a ringdown artifact with high intensity is seen around the IVUS catheter

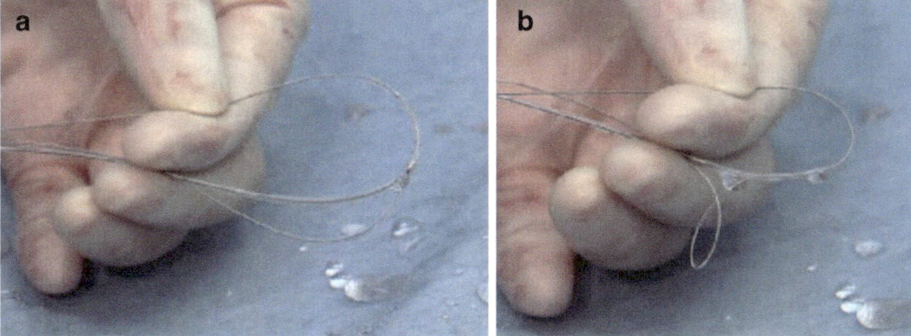

Fig. 2 Guidewire entanglement. (**a**) In highly angulated vessels, withdrawal of a tip-short monorail catheter results in misalignment of the trajectory between the catheter and the guidewire. (**b**) If you continue to pull out with a misaligned trajectory, the guidewire will be kinked at the tip of the guiding catheter, creating resistance. If the guidewire is pulled out forcibly, it will be bent

2 Entanglement of IVUS Catheter and Guidewire (Fig. 2)

The tip of the IVUS catheter may become entangled in the guidewire and be caught in the tip of the guiding catheter, making removal difficult.

2.1 Cause

Especially at sites with strong angulation, such as left circumflex artery or proximal right coronary artery, the IVUS catheter tries to return straight to the guiding catheter, whereas the guidewire does not follow it and deflects. Therefore, there is a gap in the trajectory between the IVUS catheter and the guidewire (guidewire separation, Fig. 2a), and if the guidewire is withdrawn without being noticed, the guidewire is bent and entangled at the tip of the guiding catheter (Fig. 2b).

2.2 Countermeasures

If the guidewire is entangled, you will feel some resistance during withdrawal of the IVUS catheter, so be sure to check fluoroscopy and remove both the IVUS catheter and guidewire together.

2.3 Prevention

Advice
When removing the IVUS catheter, slowly pull it out while checking the trajectory of the guidewire under fluoroscopic guidance. If the guidewire is deflected, pull the IVUS catheter out alternately while pulling the guidewire slightly forward.

In some cases, the IVUS catheter may become stuck in the distal portion of the stent and be difficult to remove (IVUS stuck).

In rare cases, an IVUS catheter may become stuck at the edge of an implanted stent and be difficult to remove. In this case, an operator is often in a panic, and it is desirable that the staff in the Cath lab be able to calmly instruct an operator on how to respond.

2.4 Cause

1. The exit port of the IVUS catheter is damaged and split finely, and a stent strut enters directly into it.
2. A gap between the IVUS catheter and the guidewire (wire separation), where the stent strut becomes entangled. This can be exacerbated by the fact that the exit port can be easily damaged by excessive force.

3. Underexpansion of the stent (especially in small vessels).
4. When the distal edge of the stent is placed in angulated segments.
5. When a stent is placed across ectatic or aneurysmal segments, it is trapped because of malapposition of the stent at the site of ectasia or aneurysma.
6. Observation of a side branch with an electronic scan IVUS catheter (Philips) through stent struts.

2.5 *How to Deal with (Problem, Etc.)*

Pay Attention Here

If you feel any discomfort or resistance, never pull the IVUS catheter any further.

Forcible withdrawal can lead to further deterioration of the stent, including shortening and deformation.

1. After confirming that the imaging core has returned to the tip, push the entire IVUS catheter in, rotate the catheter itself, and slowly pull it out again in a way that changes the location of the exit port. Repeat several times, rotating and stopping the imaging core.
2. If a 7-Fr or larger guiding catheter is used, pass the balloon catheter through the guidewire on which the IVUS catheter rests and bring it to the distal end of the stent. Push the balloon catheter into the guidewire and remove the IVUS catheter and balloon catheter. It is not necessary to dilate the balloon at this time.
3. With AltaView®· turn and remove the screw at the base of the catheter, and with OptiCross™· cut the outer tube of the IVUS catheter at the proximal part (Fig. 3a), and pull the imaging core out completely (Fig. 3b). From there, insert a RADIFOCUS® guidewire (0.021 inch or less for AltaView® and 0.025 inch or less for OptiCross™) or a PCI guidewire from the stiff end (Fig. 3c), push the entire catheter in again, rotate it to change direction, and pull it out (Fig. 3d).
4. Similarly, cut the outer sleeve of the IVUS catheter, insert the guidewire, push it into the distal part of the stent using the child catheter, remove the stuck, and pull out the entire IVUS catheter. Insert a guidewire of regular length when using a monorail-type child catheter (GuideLiner or Guidezilla™), or a 300-cm guidewire when using an ST01 or similar catheter.
5. In proximal right coronary arteries, for example, push the guiding catheter in on itself to remove the IVUS catheter.
6. Approach the site of the stack using a different system and attempt to dislodge the stuck using another guidewire or balloon. In this case, if a guiding catheter of 6 Fr or less is used, puncture another site and use another system.

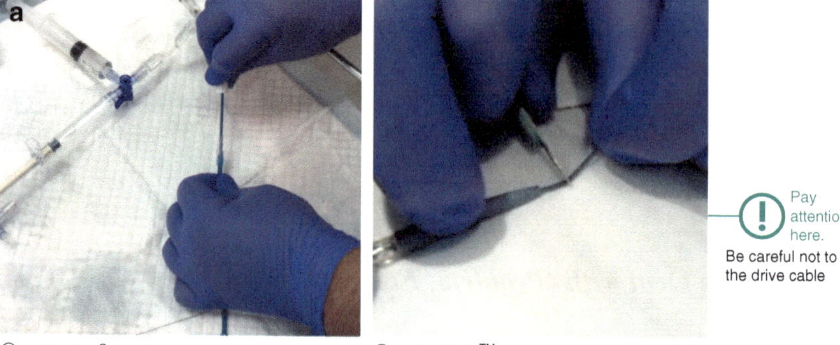

① In AltaView®, turn the screw at hand to remove it. ② In OptiCross™, the outer sheath of the IVUS catheter is cut with a scalpel.

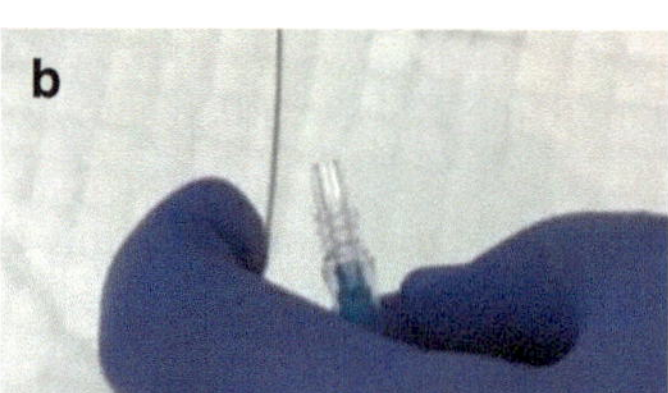

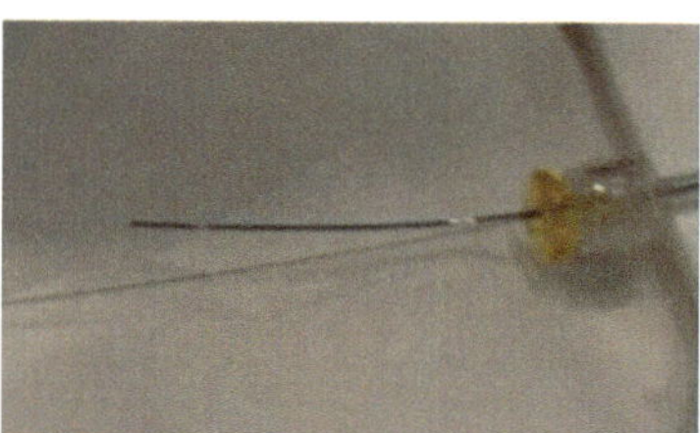

When the imaging core is withdrawn all the way to the tip, the outer sleeve of the IVUS catheter becomes a hollow tube.

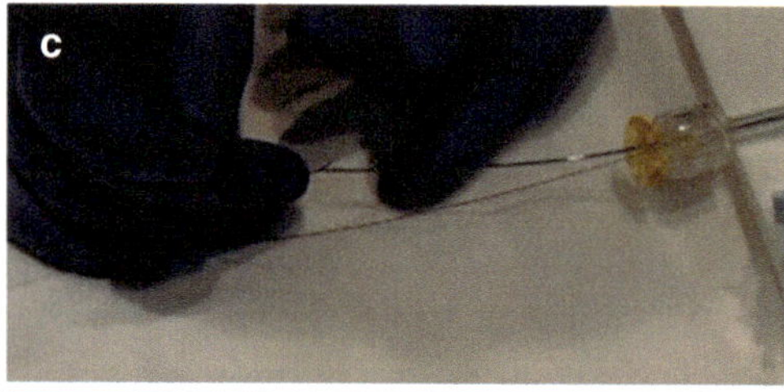

Insert a RADIFOCUS® guidewire into the outer sheath of the IVUS catheter and advance it until it cannot be pushed any further.

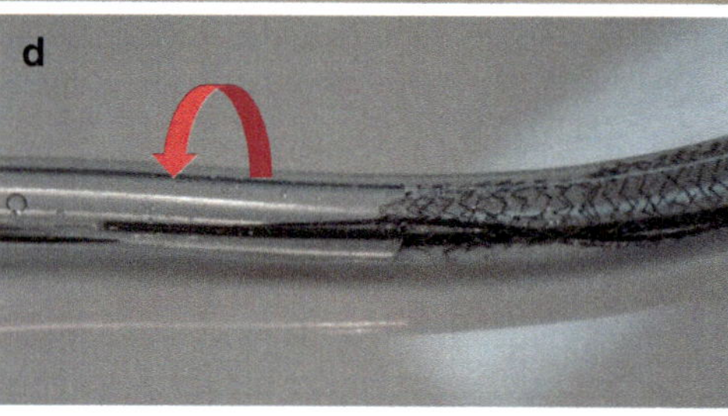

Push and turn the entire IVUS catheter slightly, and remove the IVUS catheter when it is unstuck at the tip.

Fig. 3 Removal of stacked IVUS catheter. (**a**) 1. In AltaView®· turn the screw at hand to remove it. 2. in OptiCross™, the outer sheath of the IVUS catheter is cut with a scalpel. Pay attention here. Be careful not to cut the drive cable. (**b**) When the imaging core is withdrawn all the way to the tip, the outer sleeve of the IVUS catheter becomes a hollow tube. (**c**) Insert a RADIFOCUS® guidewire into the outer sheath of the IVUS catheter and advance it until it cannot be pushed any further. (**d**) Push and turn the entire IVUS catheter slightly, and remove the IVUS catheter when it is unstuck at the tip

2.6 *Prevention*

At the end of the pullback, the imaging core has come to the proximal segment inside of the outer sheath. If an operator removes the IVUS catheter as it is, the exit port of the guidewire may get caught in the stent strut or the guidewire may become entangled at the guiding catheter tip because of the lack of stiffness at the tip. Therefore, after completion of the pullback, the imaging core should be returned to the catheter tip and removed under fluoroscopy with rotating the imaging core. Rotating the imaging core prevents the catheter tip from getting caught on the stent edge.

Excessive speed of withdrawal may cause this problem. If the guidewire is deflected, pull out the IVUS catheter alternately while pulling out the guidewire slightly forward.

Pay Attention Here

The most important thing is for the operator to remain calm and not become overwhelmed. This phenomenon can occur with all IVUS catheters marketed in Japan, and if information is promptly collected through the manufacturer and appropriate measures are taken, it will not lead to a serious situation. It goes without saying that the correct use of IVUS catheters is the best defense.

Advice

Troubleshooting videos (see YouTube).

For more information on troubleshooting IVUS catheters, we have uploaded a video to YouTube.

YouTube (https://www.youtube.com/) → Search for "IVUS Troubleshooting."

References

1. Hausmann D, et al. The safety of intracoronary ultrasound: a multicenter survey of 2207 examinations. Circulation. 1995;91:623–530.
2. Verstraete SF, et al. Acute occlusion of the left main coronary artery following intracoronary ultrasound examination. Catheter Cardiovasc Interv. 1999;47:181–4.
3. Wiyono SA, et al. Thrombotic complication during intracoronary imaging. Neth Heart J. 2012;20:229–31.

IVUS-Guided PCI Procedures and Methods

Takumi Kimura and Yoshihiro Morino

Points for Comprehensive Use

- IVUS should be performed before and after PCI to compare those findings.
- The most useful information for determining the device diameter is the reference segment, not the lesion. To determine the device length, it is important to find the segments with a residual plaque area of less than 50% as soon as possible.
- When performing marking technique, know the exact position of the IVUS transducer and the position of the balloon marker for stent implantation. The direction of CAG should be such that the lesion appears as long as possible.
- In determining the endpoint, the target lesion should be observed from sufficiently distal to proximal to the lesion. IVUS images should be reviewed for probable complications from immediately after the treatment to late phase.
- Various off-line measurements should be performed before finishing the procedure to determine the endpoint.

Supplementary Information The online version contains supplementary material available at https://doi.org/10.1007/978-981-19-5658-4_13.

T. Kimura (✉) · Y. Morino
Department of Cardiology, Division of Internal Medicine, Iwate Medical University, Morioka, Iwate, Japan
e-mail: kimutaku1119@yahoo.co.jp

J. Honye (ed.), *Basics of Comprehensive IVUS-Guided PCI*,
https://doi.org/10.1007/978-981-19-5658-4_13

1 Determination of Stent Implantation Segments and Stent Size

In the era of bare metal stent (BMS), excessive full lesion coverage was not recommended because stent length was an independent contributor to in-stent restenosis. Therefore, "spot stenting" was widely accepted for stenting diffuse lesions.

With the advent of drug-eluting stent (DES), its effectiveness in preventing restenosis has led to the need for a different PCI strategy than that of BMS. As reflected in the phrase "longer is better," the benefit of full lesion coverage in diffuse lesions has increased, and the length of stent used per lesion has clearly increased compared with the BMS era.

On the other hand, since stent length is reported to be associated with stent thrombosis and late in-stent restenosis [1, 2], excessive margins are not recommended. Of course, it is no exaggeration to say that to decide landing zones and stent size is crucial in PCI because a metal stent, once implanted, remains in a patients' body for a lifetime.

In this section, we describe how IVUS can be used to determine stent diameter and length based on our experience.

Here's the Trick

Once IVUS has passed through the lesion, an orientation should be made with reference to the stenosis and bifurcation. Use coronary angiography (CAG) to determine location of the stenosis and its relationship to the bifurcation, and keep them in mind before imaging. Especially in case of the anterior descending artery, it is easier to obtain an orientation if position of the left circumflex branch is well understood on IVUS in advance.

1.1 How to Determine the Stent Length?

DES is a device that reduces the likelihood of in-stent restenosis in the covered area.

Therefore, it is generally better to cover the whole lesion rather than leave it, which improves the clinical outcome.

However, coronary artery lesions in clinical practice are not easy to cover without leaving a lesion. When there is some degree of plaque continuity in the reference area, some kind of index is required to determine where to place the stent.

The authors use 3-step criteria (Table 1, Fig.1) to determine the optimal landing zones for DES implantation [3]. If the criteria are met up to step 2, they are optimal landing zones. To achieve this, a cutoff of 50% for the residual plaque is used. Even if the actual cross-sectional area of the reference cannot be calculated, it can be determined at a glance by remembering the sense of the plaque volume of 40–60% in Fig. 1.

Table 1 IVUS criteria for good stent positioning

Step 1. Basically, landing zones are normal segments without plaque.
Step 2. If step 1 is difficult, landing zones should be segments where plaque burden is less than 50%.
Step 3. If step 2 is also difficult, landing zones should be segments with least plaque burden.

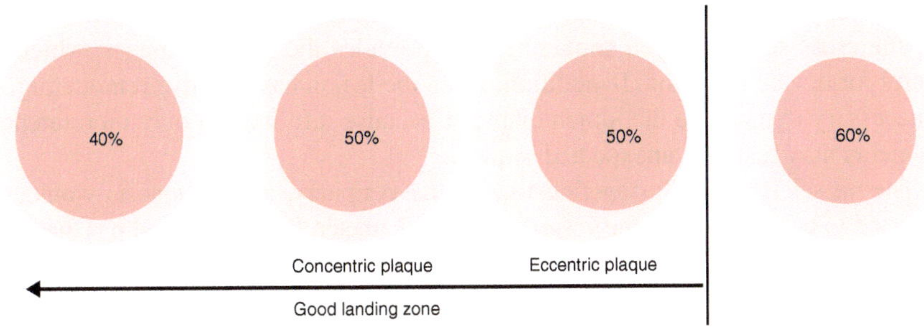

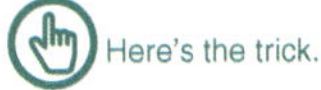

By referring plaque burden less than 50% illustrated in Fig. 1, it is possible to visually estimate landings zones.

Fig. 1 Stepwise theory for stent edge determination in DES implantation. Concentric plaque; Eccentric plaque; Good landing zone. Here's the Trick. By referring plaque burden less than 50% illustrated in Fig. 1, it is possible to visually estimate landings zones

You are able to understand that this indicator is reasonable from the fact that the reference residual plaque area is less than 50% in many DES trials.

Here's the Trick
A lesion is defined as "the area with the tightest stenosis," and in the case of diffuse lesions as "the segment with the most plaque."

1.2 How to Determine the Stent Diameter?

To determine the stent diameter, it is first necessary to obtain overall IVUS images of the planned implantation site.

1. Easy to dilate (calcification, fibrous plaque).
2. Plaque distribution.
3. Degree of vascular remodeling.
4. Are distal segments smaller than it should be due to lack of blood flow?
5. Are there any signs that may predict complications (e.g., distal emboli, perforation, and side branch occlusion)?

It is important to make a habit of observing these information so that it can be understood at the time of initial pullback. It is also important to review those images unless operators missed any findings.

To determine the stent diameter, IVUS measurements are first required to obtain cross-sectional area of the distal and proximal references (Fig. 2). Measurement of cross-sectional area is not necessary to determine the stent diameter; information on the maximum and minimum diameters is sufficient. However, it is true that measuring the cross-sectional area simultaneously provides the mean diameter, which is useful for device selection. In addition, when the lesion has negative remodeling, it is necessary to measure the lumen diameter because information only on reference segments may result in unexpected sequelae.

The vessel is naturally tapering toward the periphery, and a stenosis would be expected to be smaller than the vessel's original diameter. If there are findings that predict perforation or distal embolization, a smaller size of the device should be selected.

Pay Attention Here
The distal and proximal references are the segments with largest lumen within 10 mm of the lesion and not necessarily the segments with the least plaque.

EEM and lumen: measurement of maximum and minimum diameters

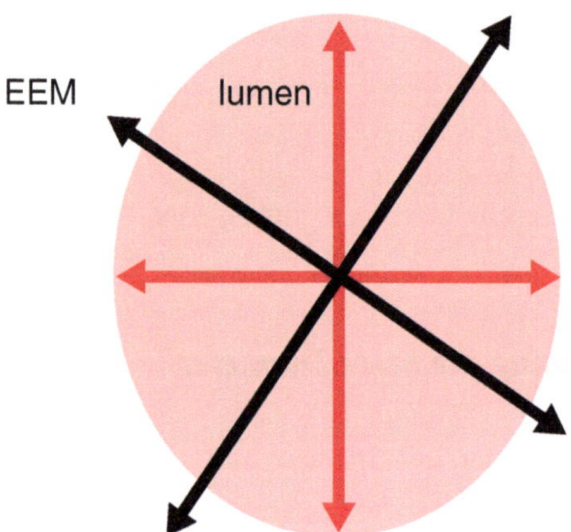

Fig. 2 Measurements required during stenting: measurement of the lumen at the reference segment. EEM and lumen: Measurement of maximum and minimum diameters. I want to know the average diameter of the lumen. 1. Estimate the average diameter from the maximum and minimum diameters. It is also possible to determine the average diameter by measuring the cross-sectional area. 2. Using mean lumen diameter. A balloon (stent) size equal to or slightly larger than the mean lumen diameter at the proximal or distal reference, whichever is smaller, was considered. Dilating to the mean diameter of the EEM increases the risk of dissection and perforation. Smaller diameter is unavoidable if there is a risk of perforation. Lumen

As you know, late loss has become negligible with DES, and the idea of covering plaque with a stent as much as possible has been combined with the idea of matching the lumen of the reference segments. Needs to take risks associated with dilatation, such as edge dissection, hematoma, and vessel perforation, are reduced compared to BMS.

Therefore, for DES with low late loss, it is recommended to select a device based on the reference lumen diameter. Specifically, maximum and minimum lumen diameters are measured and the mean lumen diameter is estimated. A balloon (stent) size with a lumen diameter equal to or slightly larger than that would be a good choice. Of course, if there is a risk of perforation, a smaller device is unavoidable.

2 Marking Technique

The purpose of marking technique with IVUS is to reduce geographic miss through accurate stenting. Marking technique is particularly important in the left main trunk, proximal anterior descending artery, and ostial right coronary artery, where shift of a stent can result in significant protrusion into the aorta and risk of side branch occlusion. Another important point is to reduce the risk of stent edge dissection and hematoma caused by geographic miss.

Marking technique may also have the advantage of reducing the amount of contrast medium used and the radiation dose to the patient, and is useful for patients with renal dysfunction and heart failure, which are increasing in the aging society.

2.1 Marking Technique in Practice

It is important to evaluate the lesion before PCI to determine whether direct stenting or predilatation is necessary. The IVUS catheter should put into sufficiently distal to the lesion and pull the transducer to an assumed segment for distal landing zone. The IVUS longitudinal measurements are then reset to zero and perform CAG using contrast as an assumed distal landing zone. The transducer is then slowly pulled back, and takes CAG again for marking an assumed proximal stent landing zone. If an IVUS catheter is not firmly fixed, the measurement in the longitudinal direction may be shifted, so care should be taken. After marking the proximal landing zone, return the transducer to the distal landing zone to confirm that the measurement for stent length is correct.

Because the position of the transducer differs among IVUS companies, it is important to know the exact position of the transducer before use (details are omitted). In addition, there are three types of stents in which the balloon marker is mounted: one on the inside, one in the middle, and one on the outside of the stent.

CAG should be performed in a direction that allows the lesion to be visualized as long as possible (long-axis CAG). If the flat panel is placed too far cranial or caudal, the lesion may be shortened, although the bifurcation may be well visualized. It is important to note that slight differences in markings technique may be difficult to recognize. If possible, CAG should be taken from at least two directions during marking technique to reduce geographic miss (Fig. 3).

a: IVUS marking of the proximal anterior descending artery

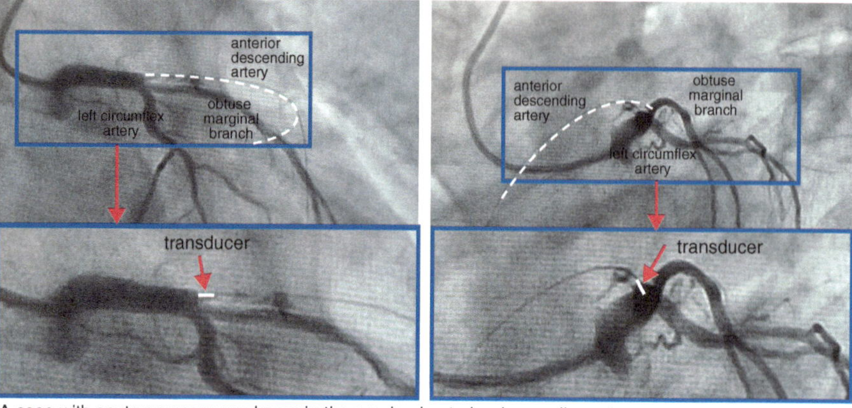

A case with acute coronary syndrome in the proximal anterior descending artery.
We used IVUS to mark stent landing zones in the most proximal part of the anterior descending artery (distal to the circumflex and obtuse marginal branch) considering the difference in vessel diameter and angle of bifurcation.

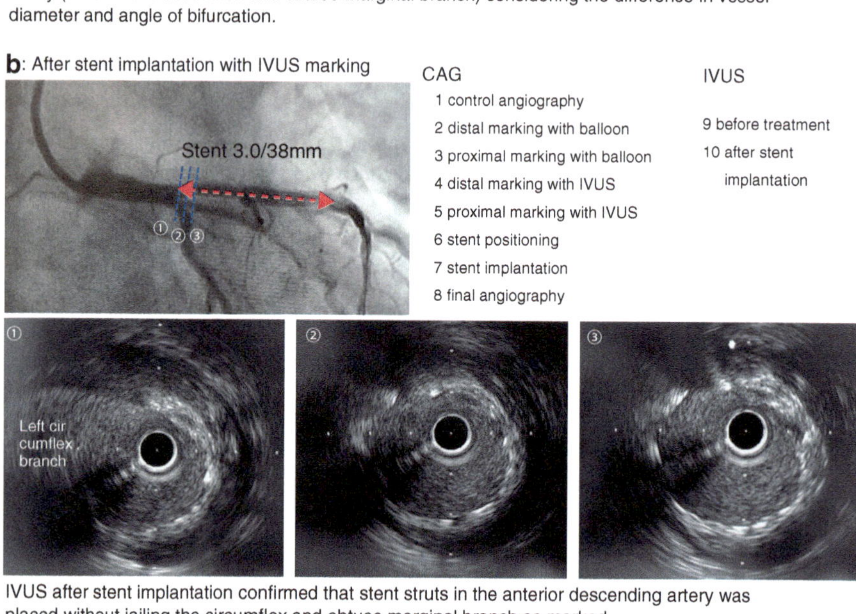

IVUS after stent implantation confirmed that stent struts in the anterior descending artery was placed without jailing the circumflex and obtuse marginal branch as marked.

Fig. 3 Actual marking technique. (**a**) IVUS marking of the proximal anterior descending artery. A case with acute coronary syndrome in the proximal anterior descending artery. We used IVUS to mark stent landing zones in the most proximal part of the anterior descending artery (distal to the circumflex and obtuse marginal branch) considering the difference in vessel diameter and angle of bifurcation. Anterior descending artery; Left circumflex artery; Obtuse marginal branch; Transducer. (**b**) After stent implantation with IVUS marking. IVUS after stent implantation confirmed that stent struts in the anterior descending artery were placed without jailing the circumflex and obtuse marginal branch as marked. Stent 3.0/38 mm; Left circumflex branch. Video available (Videos S1–S10). IVUS marking case (different case from Fig. 3). CAG: 1. control angiography; 2. distal marking with balloon; 3. proximal marking with balloon; 4. distal marking with IVUS; 5. proximal marking with IVUS; 6. stent positioning; 7. stent implantation; 8. final angiography. · IVUS: 9. before treatment; 10. after stent implantation

The marking technique is also useful in chronic total occlusive (CTO) lesions, where it is possible to find the entry point with marking technique when a side branch emerges from a presumed occlusion.

Here's the Trick
Marking technique for the bifurcation of left anterior descending artery and left circumflex artery should be performed with spider view (LAO, CAU) and the right anterior oblique caudal projection (RAO, CAU). Marking of the ostial left main trunk should be performed from the anterior cranial position (AP, CRA) or from the anterior slight left cranial oblique projection (AP, LAO).

LAO: Left anterior oblique.
CAU: Caudal.
RAO: Right anterior oblique.
AP: Anteroposterior.
CRA: CRANIAL.

Pay Attention Here
When measuring and marking length of the lesion by moving an IVUS transducer, it is important to note that if the IVUS catheter itself is displaced, lesion length and marking positions will be displaced if it is performed from a distal to proximal segment. For confirmation, check the lesion length again from a proximal to distal segment to reduce errors.

3 Endpoint Determination

In Japan, the use of IVUS during PCI is currently reimbursed by insurance, and it can be used regardless of complexity of the lesion. The era of angiography (angiography-guided) PCI has been changing to the era of IVUS-guided PCI. In recent years, optical coherence tomography (OCT)-guided PCI has also been performed. Of course, the resolution of angiographic guidance is limited in assessing intravascular microstructural changes and stent expansion.

Although there have been many studies of angiography-guided versus IVUS-guided PCI, IVUS-guided procedures have been shown to significantly reduce major cardiovascular events (MACE), especially in long lesions, left main trunk, bifurcation, and CTO lesions. This is largely due to a reduction in target vessel revascularization, and IVUS guidance has been reported to reduce stent thrombosis and cardiac death. Therefore, it is important to determine the endpoint of IVUS-guided procedures, and here we will discuss the endpoint of IVUS in the setting of DES implantation.

3.1 Determination of IVUS Endpoints

When IVUS is performed after stent implantation, it is recommended that the IVUS catheter be brought sufficiently distal to the stent and observed proximally with automatic pullback. In some cases, it is difficult to put the IVUS catheter to the distal portion of the stent, especially in small or tortuous vessels, however, these lesions are more likely to have stent underexpansion or distal edge dissection, so observation is necessary.

In recent years, some IVUS systems have faster pullback speeds than previous systems, making it difficult to determine the endpoint of stent implantation in real time. Therefore, it is important to perform an automatic pullback first, and then reobserve manually the stent and the reference segments. It is recommended that IVUS review be completed before the procedure is completely finished so that the minimum stent area (MSA) the residual plaque area should be measured, and post-dilation or additional stent implantation can be considered if necessary. After stenting, IVUS should be performed at distal to the stent, in-stent, and proximal to the stent, respectively, to minimize oversight. The main segments of observation and their contents are shown in Fig. 4.

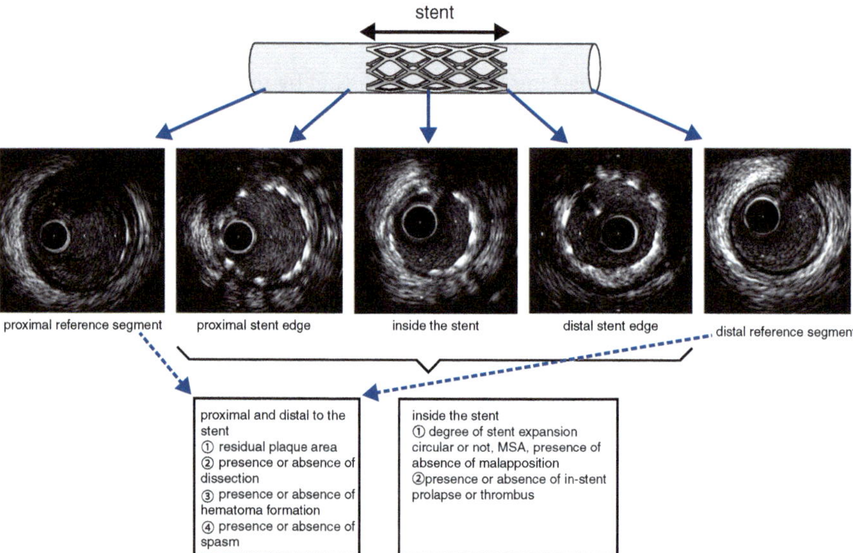

Fig. 4 Main observation points after stent implantation. Stent; proximal reference segment; proximal stent edge; inside the stent; distal stent edge; distal reference segment; proximal and distal to the stent. 1. residual plaque area; 2. presence or absence of dissection; 3. presence or absence of hematoma formation; 4. presence or absence of spasm. Inside the stent. 1. degree of stent expansion. MSA, malapposition, circular or not, MSA, presence of absence of malapposition. 2. presence or absence of in-stent prolapse or thrombus

3.2 Distal and Proximal to the Stent

In DES era, treatment is directed toward full coverage of the plaque. Because coronary arteries are generally tapered toward the periphery, it is not feasible to treat long lesions with a single stent. Therefore, when difference in vessel diameter between distal and proximal segments is large, it is necessary to use two stents.

When the decision is made to use a single stent, diameter of the stent is determined according to the distal reference vessel, but an oversized stent may still be placed. What occurs there is distal dissection and associated hematoma formation. Small dissections may be missed by IVUS, and deep dissections that extend to the tunica media may extend distally and induce ischemia, so additional stent implantation should be considered (Fig. 5).

Hematomas are usually created in the absence of reentry after dissection, and at first glance on IVUS, echogenicity of hematoma is quite similar to fibrous plaques, so care should be taken not to miss them. In the distal part of the stent, progressive dissection is more likely to occur, resulting in coronary occlusion. We need to pay attention to the tissue outside the coronary artery. Coronary artery perforation may be observed on IVUS (Fig. 6), and if contrast leakage is feared, it is necessary to identify the site of perforation and treat it with IVUS guidance.

Although dissection and hematoma formation are relatively rare in proximal segments to the stent, there is a possibility of stent underexpansion, which should be evaluated by IVUS. Care should be taken to ensure that no oversight is made at the end of procedure, as post-dilation may cause a balloon to interfere with the proximal segment, causing dissection and hematoma formation. Retrograde dissection is more likely to occur in segments proximal to the stent than in the distal part, and although it is less likely to lead to coronary occlusion, additional stenting should be considered if there is extensive dissection in large vessels.

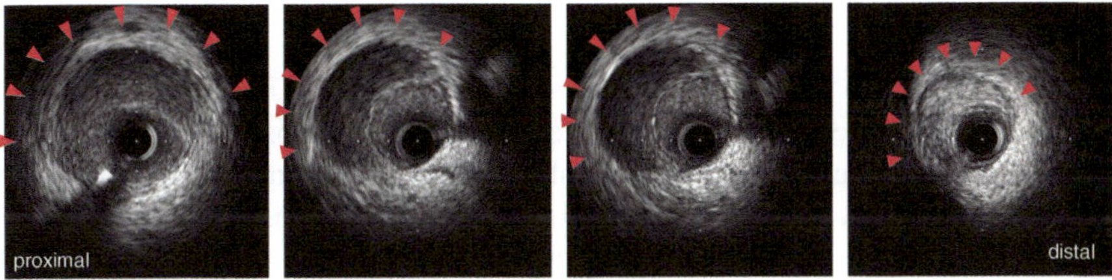

Fig. 5 Hematoma formation distal to the stent. There was hematoma formation at the distal end of the stent. The distal part of the stent was found to be compressed by the hematoma, and an additional stent was implanted. Proximal; Distal

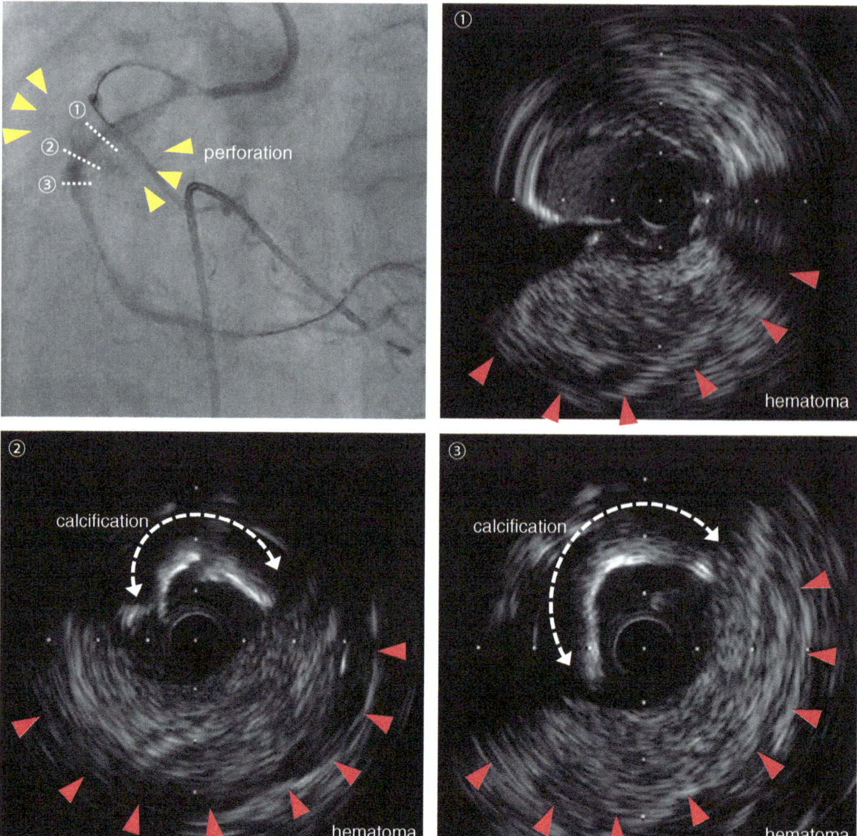

Fig. 6 Coronary artery perforation confirmed by IVUS. When IVUS was performed after POBA to a calcified lesion in right coronary artery, a large hematoma was observed and the diagnosis of coronary artery perforation was made. Perforation; Hematoma; Calcification

3.3 In-Stent

The inside of the stent should be observed for circular expansion, for plaque prolapse inside of the stent, and for any thrombus or hematoma formation. Measurement of MSA is essential, as is the presence of malapposition of the stent (Fig. 7). Blood speckles outside the stent strut are also important.

In the era of BMS, late lumen loss was large and the MSA was obtained as large as possible to reduce restenosis and post-PCI ischemic events. However, in the era of DES, restenosis was less common and late lumen loss varied among stent types, and there are no criteria for stent expansion. However, there is a report [4] that a larger MSA than cross-sectional area in the distal reference segment can reduce revascularization.

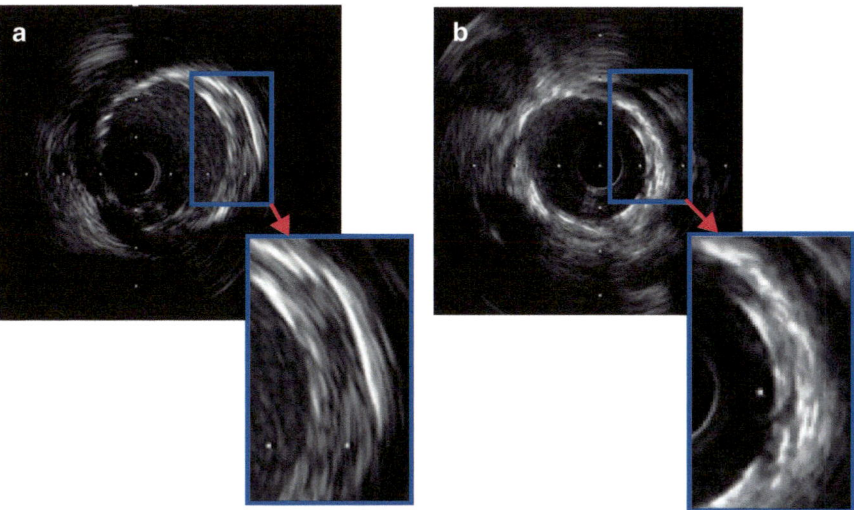

Fig. 7 Confirmation of blood speckles outside stent struts. (**a**) Blood speckles were observed outside stent struts and post-dilation was performed with a diagnosis of malapposition. (**b**) There were no blood speckles outside stent struts, and post-dilation was determined unnecessary

Here's the Trick
When observing outside of the stent struts or when the boundary of neointima is unclear, flushing with heparinized saline (negative contrast) or contrast medium (positive contrast) can remove blood speckles and clarify the boundary.

Pay Attention Here
In particular, small dissections and hematomas at both ends of the stent may be missed without careful observation, and an operator should review again after high-speed pullback. If there is a possibility for compression of true lumen, it is important not to remove the guidewire, and to observe it again by IVUS after a period of time.

References

1. Fujii K, Carlier SG, Mintz GS, et al. Stent underexpansion and residual reference segment stenosis are related to stent thrombosis after sirolimus-eluting stent implantation: an intravascular ultrasound study. J Am Coll Cardiol. 2005;45:995–8.
2. Moreno R, Fernández C, Hernández R, et al. Drug-eluting stent thrombosis: results from a pooled analysis including 10 randomized studies. J Am Coll Cardiol. 2005;45:954–9.
3. Morino Y, Tamiya S, Masuda N, et al. Intravascular ultrasound criteria for determination of optimal longitudinal positioning of sirolimus-eluting stents. Circ J. 2010;74:1609–16.
4. Hong SJ, Kim BK, Shin DH, et al. Effect of intravascular ultrasound-guided vs angiography- guided everolimus-eluting stent implantation: the IVUS- XPL randomized clinical trial. JAMA. 2015;314:2155–63.

Tips for Stentless PCI

Tomoko Kobayashi

> **Points for Comprehensive Utilization**
> - Determination of PCI strategy based on plaque characteristics.
> - Evaluation of acquired lumen area and residual plaque occupancy.
> - Presence and/or absence of dissection and its morphology, complications of hematoma, and risk assessment for acute coronary occlusion.

With improved results of drug-eluting stents (DES), stentless PCI is an option only in a limited number of patients. These include patients for release of ischemia before surgical treatment, patients who require concomitant anticoagulants for atrial fibrillation, and younger patients who want to avoid stenting. Conventional balloon therapy alone is associated with a high rate of restenosis, but use of drug-coated balloons (DCBs) has improved results and indication is expanding. Because of the risk of acute coronary occlusion with stentless PCI, endpoint determination using intravascular imaging is safer.

T. Kobayashi (✉)
Department of Internal Medicine, Cardiovascular Center, Kyoto Katsura Hospital, Nishikyo-ku, Kyoto, Japan
e-mail: kcvc.kobayashi@katsura.com

J. Honye (ed.), *Basics of Comprehensive IVUS-Guided PCI*,
https://doi.org/10.1007/978-981-19-5658-4_14

1 PCI Strategies According to Vessel Diameter and Presence of Calcium

1.1 *Stentless PCI for Non-calcified Small Vessels (Reference Vessel Diameter < 2.8 mm) with DCB (Fig. 1)*

Stentless PCI with DCB had been performed in 454 consecutive lesions since March 2014; in our hospital 73% of lesions underwent pre-dilation with scoring balloons including cutting balloons. The balloon diameter for pre-dilatation was 2.4 mm, the balloon diameter of DCB was 2.6 mm, and the dilatation pressure was 8 atm. The final dissection morphology was type A or less in 65%, type B in 23%, type C in 9%, and type D or more in 3%. Six months later, the restenosis rate was 8%, late lumen loss was −0.02 mm, and lumen enlargement was observed in 53%.

Because there is little lumen loss, imaging-based PCI strategies include (1) balloon size equivalent to the reference vessel diameter, (2) dilation pressure to minimize dissection, and (3) lumen area equivalent to the reference vessel. Therefore, a scoring balloon with the size of lumen diameter equivalent to a nearby area with least plaque occupancy should be selected, because it is able to achieve good dilatation effect with lower dilatation pressure.

1.2 *Stentless Treatment with DCB for Non-calcified Large Vessels (Control Vessel Diameter ≥ 2.8 mm) (Fig. 2)*

Directional coronary atherectomy (DCA) was revived in June 2015, and 87 lesions were treated stentless with DCB. Forty-three percent of the patients had preoperative, atrial fibrillation comorbidity, and young patient background. IVUS-guided DCA was performed to achieve residual plaque occupancy of 50%, and DCB was added after plaque removal. All cases had Type A or less dissociation. The lumen area after DCA was 6.9 mm^2 and the residual plaque occupancy was 55%, and the final lumen area after DCB was 7.7 mm^2 and the residual plaque occupancy was 52%. The restenosis rate at 6 months was 4.3%, late lumen loss was 0.31 mm, and late lumen enlargement was observed in 33%.

Because large vessels with high plaque volume have slightly higher lumen loss in the chronic phase, imaging-based PCI strategies aim for 1. lumen expansion with adequate plaque removal and 2. IVUS-guided debulking and low-pressure dilation without complications of medial dissection or hematoma.

1.3 *Stentless Treatment of Calcified Lesions (Fig. 3)*

Calcified lesions continue to contribute to restenosis after DES introduction. Rotablator and orbital atherectomy system (OAS) are effective for calcified lesions. Optical coherence tomography (OCT)/optical frequency domain imaging (OFDI)

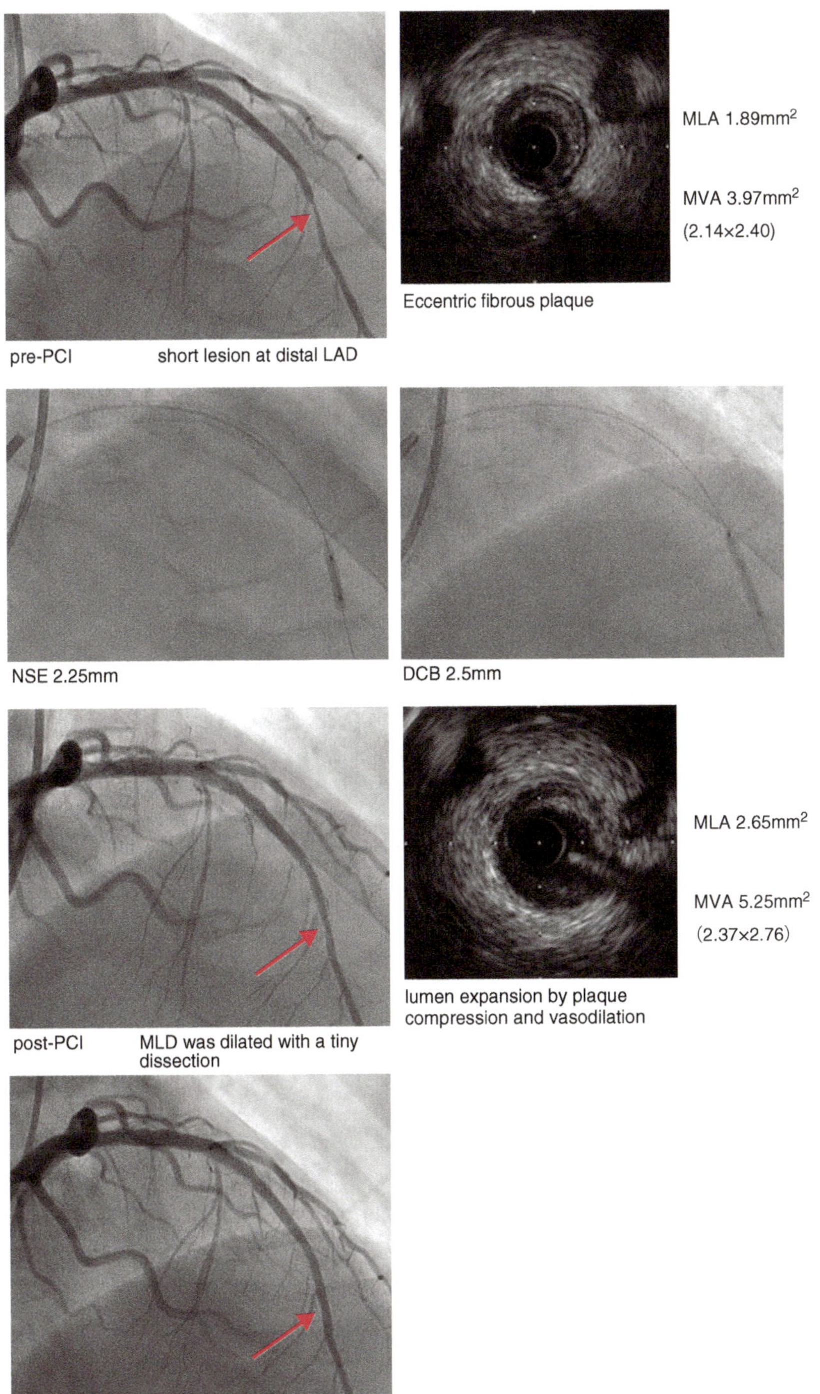

Fig. 1 Stentless PCI for non-calcified small vessel non-slip element (NSE) balloon + DCB case. Pre-PCI; IVUS showed Eccentric fibrous plaque; post-PCI; IVUS showed lumen expansion by plaque compression and vessel expansion; 6 months later

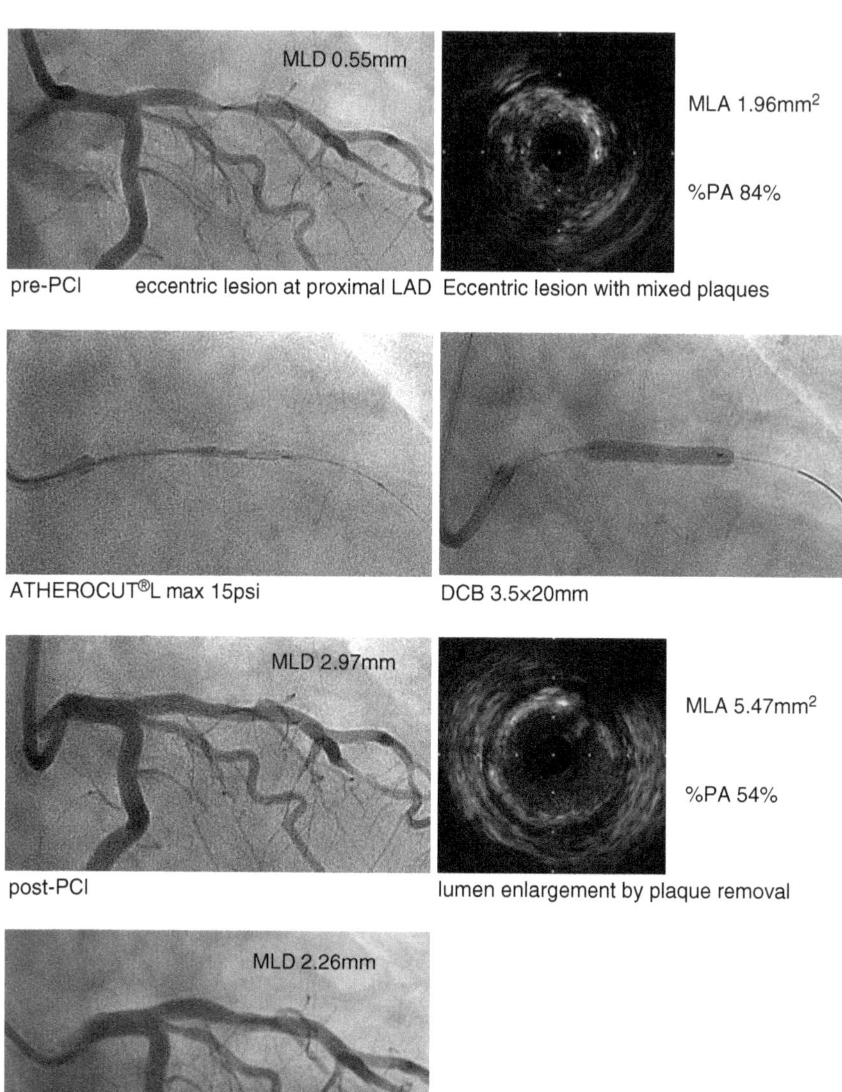

Fig. 2 Stent less PCI for non-calcified large vessel DCA + DCB case. Pre-PCI; IVUS showed Eccentric lesion with mixed plaques; post-PCI; IVUS showed lumen enlargement by plaque removal 6 months later; There was no restenosis

guidance is recommended, and intravascular imaging can be used to safely and effectively ablate calcification and expand the lumen.

Since 2016, 129 lesions underwent stentless PCI with DCB after ablating calcium by rotablator or OAS in our hospital. Imaging was used to assess wire bias and to ablate calcium whenever possible. A mean of 1.5 burrs were used, and high-speed

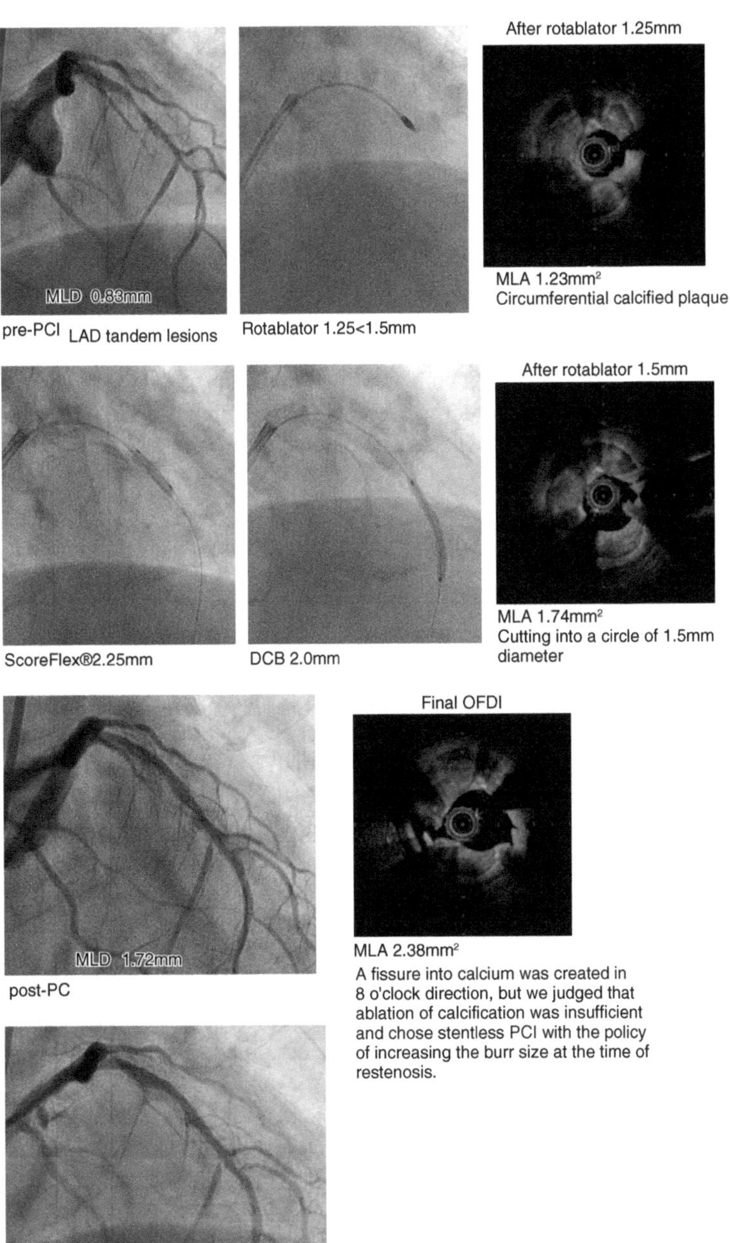

Fig. 3 Rotablator + DCB case. Pre-PCI; OFDI could not cross Rotablator 1.25 < 1.5 mm; Rotablation was performed After rotablator 1.25 mm; OFDI showed Circumferential calcified plaque; After rotablator 1.5 mm; OFDI showed Cutting into a circle of 1.5 mm diameter; post-PCI; Angiogram showed well dilated lesions. Final OFDI: OFDI showed A fissure into calcium was created in 8 o'clock direction, but we judged that ablation of calcification was insufficient and chose stentless PCI with the policy of increasing the burr size at the time of restenosis

OAS was performed in 62% of cases. Pre-dilation with a cutting/scoring balloon was performed in all patients, and DCB was added. Chronic results differed between small and large vessels. In reference vessels <2.8 mm, late lumen loss was 0.09 mm, restenosis rate 5.7%, and late lumen enlargement 49% which was quite favorable but in vessels >2.8 mm, late lumen loss was 0.28 mm, restenosis rate 13.2%, and late lumen enlargement 33%.

Although it is difficult to observe the entire vessel by imaging and to assess the amount of residual plaque, the results may be somewhat lower in large vessels because adequate ablation of calcium by available ablation devices is not possible. Imaging-based PCI strategies include (1) safe and maximal ablation of calcium and (2) low-pressure dilation using a scoring balloon of equivalent size to the reference vessel diameter. However, stent implantation significantly reduces restenosis rate (13.2% vs. 2%) in lesions with large vessels that have undergone maximal ablation and scoring modification, so PCI strategy should be determined based on the lesion and patient background.

2 Risk Assessment for Stentless PCI

Avoidance of the risk of acute coronary occlusion is an important consideration when determining the endpoint for completion of stentless PCI. Dissection findings with a high risk of acute coronary occlusion are: (1) reaching tunica media, (2) progressive hematoma formation without reentry, and (3) minimal plaque in the vessel distal to the hematoma formation site.

Figure 4 shows a case of dissection formation in a short-segment lesion with mixed eccentric calcium. Since dissection and hematoma were judged to be small and not progressing, the procedure was completed with DCB, but 3 hours later, the patient developed coronary occlusion. At the time of repeat PCI, hematoma had spread to the distal vessel that compressed the lumen. The hematoma continued to grow distally because the size of the dissection behind the calcified plaque was not adequately assessed when endpoint was determined at the time of initial procedure, there was no reentry to decompress the hematoma, and distal to the lesion was a normal vessel without plaque.

Figure 5 shows a dissection that reached media after DCA, and prolonged inflation with perfusion balloon was performed. However, there was no improvement in both dissection and hematoma, and it was judged that bailout stenting was necessary, and stentless treatment was abandoned. After DES implantation, hematoma developed in the distal vessel, but the entry was occluded, so the procedure was terminated without further development. The CAG immediately after PCI showed a stenosis in the hematoma area of the mid-LAD, the CAG next day showed a trend toward hematoma resorption.

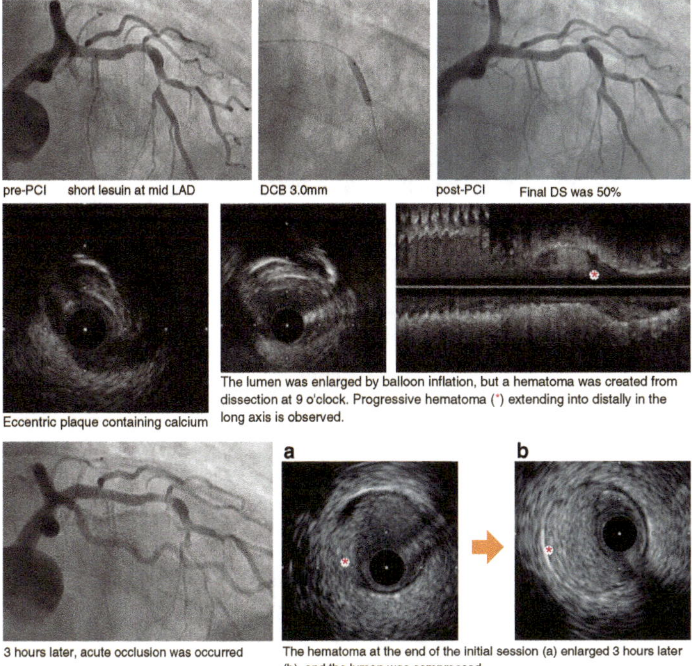

Fig. 4 Case of acute occlusion due to hematoma extension. Pre-PCI; Eccentric plaque containing calcium; post-PCI; The lumen was enlarged by balloon inflation, but a hematoma was created from dissection at 9 o'clock. Progressive hematoma (*) extending distally in the long axis is observed. 3 h later, acute occlusion was occurred. The hematoma at the end of the initial session (**a**) enlarged 3 h later (**b**), and the lumen was compressed

Here's the Trick

The final decision on whether or not a residual dissection can be terminated stentlessly is the absence of a dissection or hematoma that can develop into a blood flow obstruction and a dissection configuration that allows easy guidewire re-passage in the event of acute coronary occlusion complications. If the decision is difficult to make, it should be confirmed by temporal changes in intravascular imaging after waiting for 30 minutes.

Advice

Stentless PCI can expand indications and improve clinical outcomes by utilizing the lumen-expanding effect of plaque ablation and intimal growth inhibitory effect of DCB. Intravascular imaging is essential to confirm the efficacy and safety of PCI.

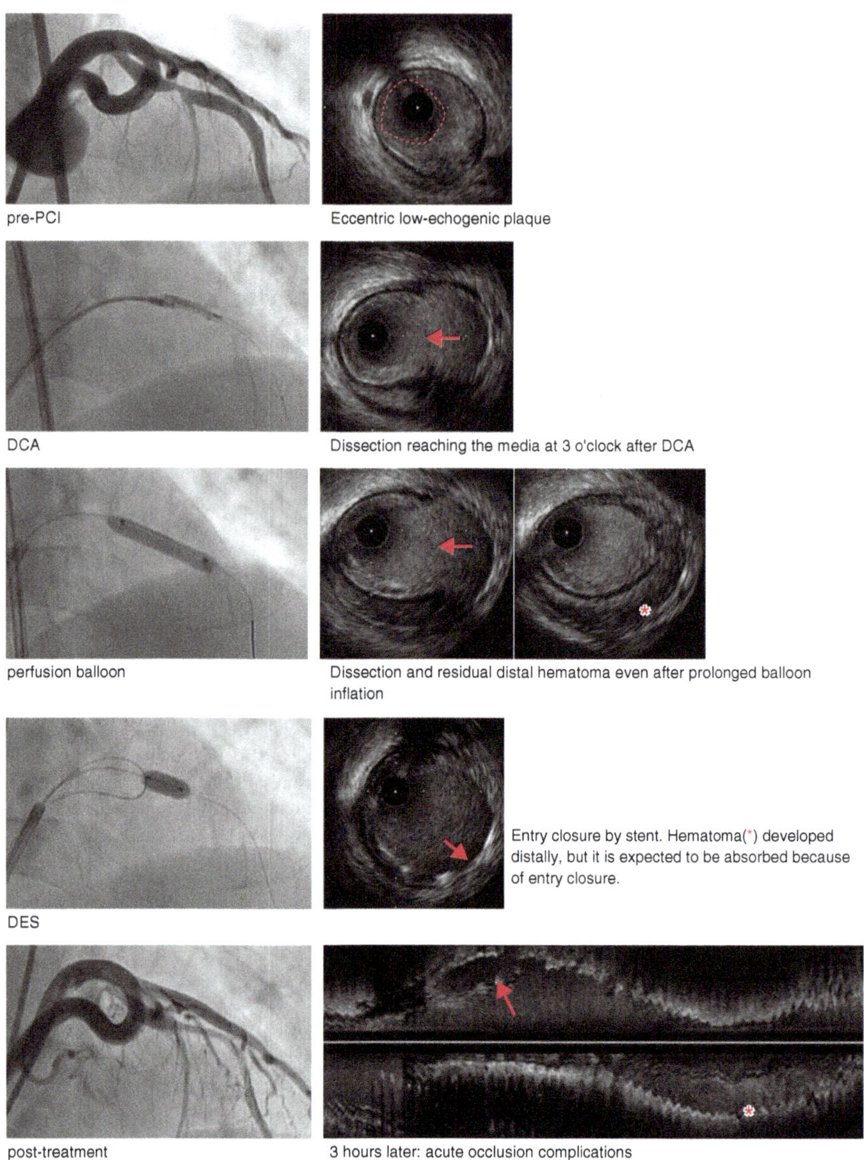

Fig. 5 Addition of stent implantation due to hematoma extension. Pre-PCI; Eccentric low-echogenic plaque. Dissociation reaching the media at 3 o'clock after DCA. Dissection and residual distal hematoma even after prolonged balloon inflation. Entry closure by stent. Hematoma(*) developed distally, but it is expected to be absorbed because of entry closure. Post-treatment

Evaluation of Thrombus and its Application to PCI

Hideki Kitahara and Yoshio Kobayashi

Points for Comprehensive Use

- Observation of thrombus with video instead of still image.
- Use of negative contrast method.
- Determination of therapeutic strategy in consideration of the pathophysiology and lesion background that led to thrombus formation.

Intracoronary thrombus is closely related to the development of acute coronary syndromes and stent thrombosis, and cannot only compromise coronary blood flow and cause myocardial ischemia and necrosis, but can also cause further expansion of the area of myocardial necrosis due to distal embolization if it is treated incorrectly. Therefore, in cases where thrombus is suspected on coronary angiography, it is important to use IVUS to evaluate thrombus and its lesion background in as much detail as possible, and to develop an appropriate PCI strategy.

1 Observation of Thrombus by IVUS

By IVUS, thrombi are observed as layered, lobulated, or pedunculated intravascular structures, typically convex toward the vessel lumen, and many of them are mobile with beating [1]. Internal echogenicity depends on the nature of thrombus

H. Kitahara · Y. Kobayashi (✉)
Department of Cardiovascular Medicine, Graduate School of Medicine, Chiba University, Chiba, Japan
e-mail: hidekita.0306@gmail.com; yuiryosuke@msn.com

J. Honye (ed.), *Basics of Comprehensive IVUS-Guided PCI*,
https://doi.org/10.1007/978-981-19-5658-4_15

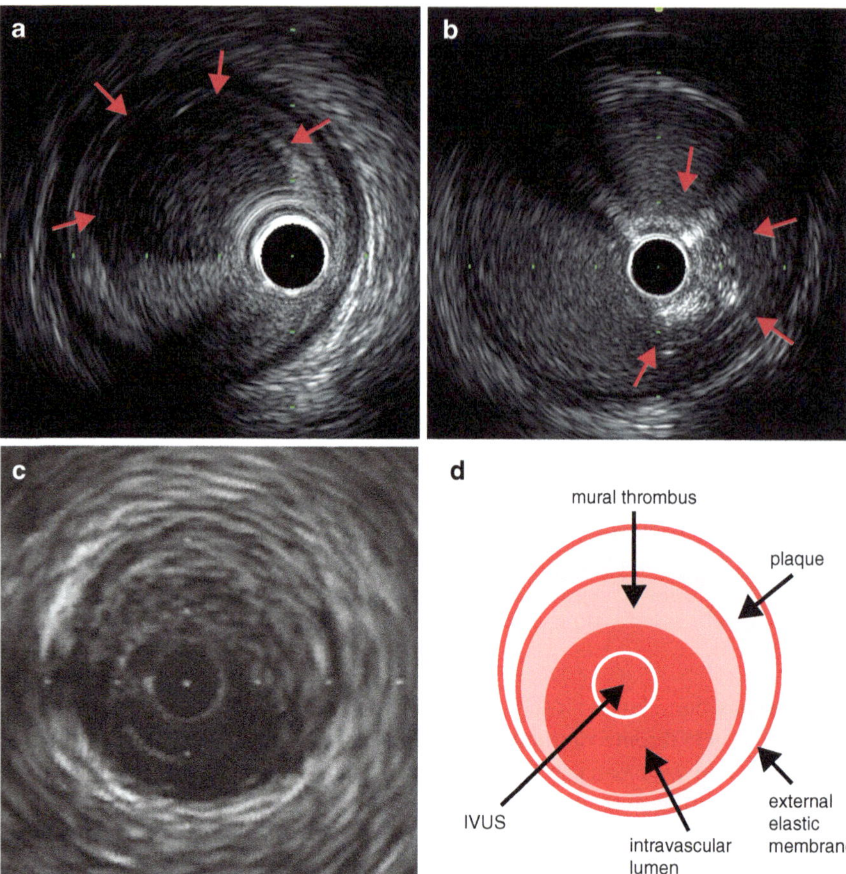

Fig. 1 Hypoechoic thrombus image suggestive of fresh thrombus (**a**: arrow), relatively hyperechoic thrombus image suggestive of organized thrombus (**b**: arrow), and mural thrombus (**c**, **d**). mural thrombus; plaque; external elastic membrane; intravascular lumen

and varies from relatively hypoechoic (newer thrombus, Fig. 1a) to hyperechoic (older thrombus, Fig. 1b). In addition, internal echo image is often spotted and granular, and blood flow through gaps and microchannels inside of the structure may be observed.

Detailed observation by video should be performed because the boundary between stagnant blood and thrombus is often indistinct and difficult to assess adequately with still images when the stenosis is tight or the structure of thrombus is complex. In such cases, the boundary with the lumen can be clearly identified by negative contrast with intracoronary injection of contrast medium or saline (Fig. 2). In addition, the boundary with the surrounding tissue is often obscured, especially for those that are not mobile, such as mural thrombi (Fig. 1c).

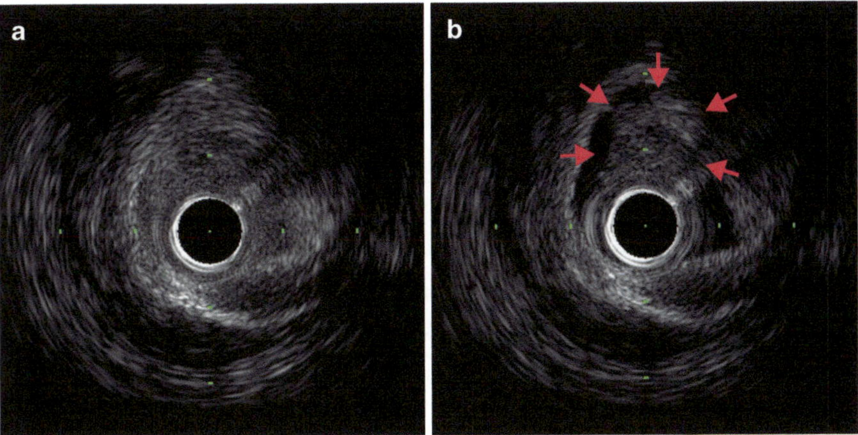

Fig. 2 An example of thrombus clearly delineated by negative contrast with contrast medium. (**a**) Thrombus without contrast medium, (**b**) thrombus with contrast medium (arrow)

2 Use of IVUS in Thrombotic Lesions

2.1 Acute Coronary Syndrome (de Novo Lesion)

In patients with acute coronary syndrome, it is important to understand pathophysiology using IVUS after securing blood flow, and to use this information for PCI. IVUS can help in the evaluation of thrombi that are difficult to identify by angiography alone, or that are diagnosed as thrombi on angiography but are actually calcification or plaque (Fig. 3).

If thrombus is identified, thrombus aspiration or use of a distal protection device may be considered, but their routine use is not recommended by the Japanese Circulation Society's Guidelines for Acute Coronary Syndromes (revised 2018) and should only be performed selectively in cases where they are likely to be effective. Mobile and unstable thrombi, massive thrombi, and hypoechoic fresh thrombi are considered to be more likely to cause distal emboli. In addition to thrombus formation, the underlying plaque condition also plays a major role in distal embolization. From Japan, it has been reported that the incidence of no-reflow phenomenon was reduced by thrombus aspiration and use of distal protection devices in patients with ultrasound-attenuated plaques of 5 mm or more in the long axis direction on IVUS2) [2]. Furthermore, this effect tended to be more remarkable in patients with an obvious thrombus. Therefore, of thrombus aspiration and distal protection devices should be considered in cases with extremely unstable tissues in which thrombus and attenuated plaque coexist. In clinical practice, however, it is often difficult to differentiate between thrombus and surrounding tissue, so it is important to understand the extent of unstable tissue including thrombus.

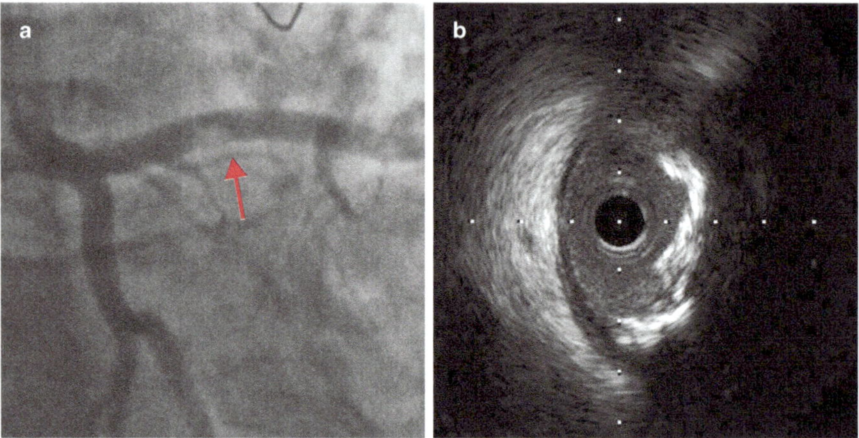

Fig. 3 Angiography showed a translucent image (**a** arrow) in the proximal LAD, which was suspected to be a thrombus, but IVUS showed a calcified lesion protruding into the lumen (**b**)

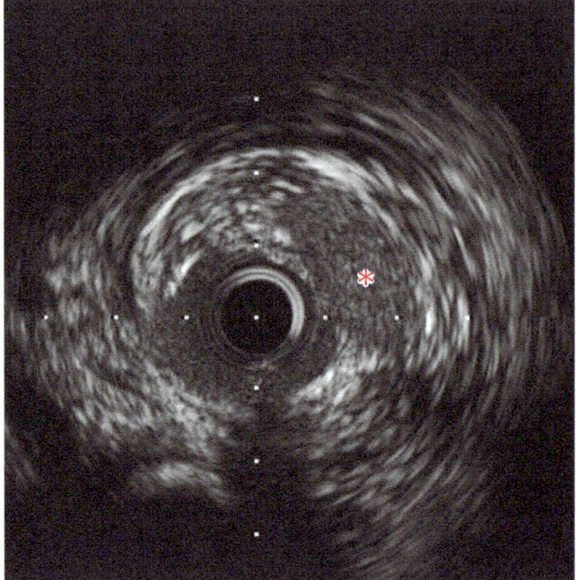

Fig. 4 Plaque disruption proximal to the culprit lesion (*)

The balloon and stent size are then determined based on the information of the lesion. In some cases, the lesion is accompanied by an unstable plaque or a plaque rupture that caused thrombus formation near the culprit lesion (Fig. 4), and appropriate stenting including these areas is performed if necessary. After stenting, IVUS is performed to evaluate stent expansion, residual stenosis, thrombus, and dissection, and additional stenting or balloon dilation is performed as needed. Additional stenting or balloon dilation should be performed if necessary. Tissue protrusion into the stent is often observed, and additional thrombus aspiration or balloon dilation should be considered if a large amount of unstable thrombus is present or blood flow is compromised. On the other hand, if the stent is sufficiently expanded and there is no obstruction to blood flow, many patients can be followed up with appropriate anticoagulants and antiplatelet agents. In addition, although rare, acute coronary syndromes may occur due to thrombosis caused by intimal erosion or coronary spasm without obvious plaque, and in this case, those patients often have good clinical course with thrombus aspiration alone [3].

[Here's the Trick] Figure out how much unstable tissue, including thrombi, is present.

2.2 *Stent Thrombosis*

Since stent thrombosis most often develops clinically as an acute coronary syndrome, the purpose of IVUS is the same as above: to evaluate thrombi, to determine the pathogenesis, and to determine PCI strategy based on the findings. Thrombus aspiration should be considered when a massive thrombus is found on IVUS, but although it contributes to the restoration of blood flow, its prognostic value has not been established [4]. If IVUS shows stent underexpansion or incomplete stent apposition, balloon dilation with an appropriate size should be performed. If dissection or stenosis of the stent edge, stent fracture, neointima, or neoatherosclerosis are observed, additional stenting is often required.

The trick is to determine the cause of thrombus formation by IVUS.

2.3 *Venous Graft Lesion*

Venous grafts with atherosclerotic changes contain large amounts of thrombus and vulnerable plaque, similar to the lesion responsible for acute coronary syndromes, and are known to be highly prone to distal embolization during PCI (Fig. 5). Therefore, distal embolization should be assumed from the beginning of the procedure. The role of IVUS here is more focused on determining stent size and procedural endpoints rather than assessing thrombotic lesions. Based on IVUS measurements, it is important to ensure adequate stent lumen and prevent excessive stent expansion.

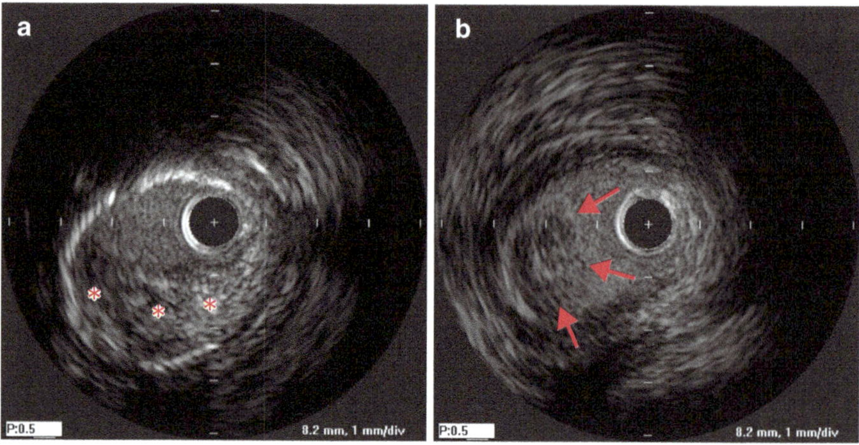

Fig. 5 Venous graft lesion with thrombus. Lesion consisting of massive thrombus and vulnerable plaque (**a***), floating thrombus (**b** arrow)

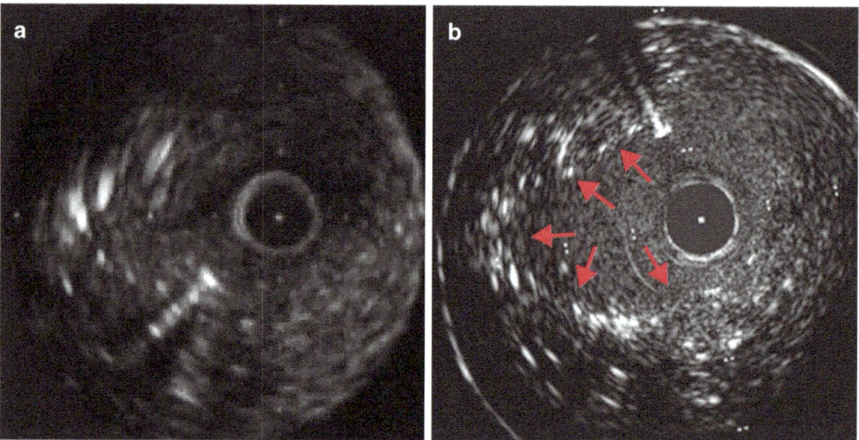

Fig. 6 Results of an experiment in which red thrombi were observed under blood flow. The thrombus was more clearly visualized with 60 MHz IVUS (**b**) than with 40 MHz IVUS (**a**) (arrows)

3 Observation of Thrombus by High-Resolution IVUS

In recent years, several high-resolution IVUS systems have been introduced that use higher frequencies than previously available. In our ex vivo experiments using a 60-MHz High-Definition IVUS system from ACIST Medical Systems, Inc., we were able to observe thrombi more clearly than with 40 MHz IVUS (Fig. 6). In addition, when we compared thrombus images in acute coronary syndromes using Terumo's AltaView® catheter with 60 MHz and 40 MHz, some thrombi were observed somewhat more clearly with 60 MHz, although there was often no significant difference (Fig. 7). In the future, it will be necessary to verify how useful this technique is for observation of thrombi in daily clinical practice.

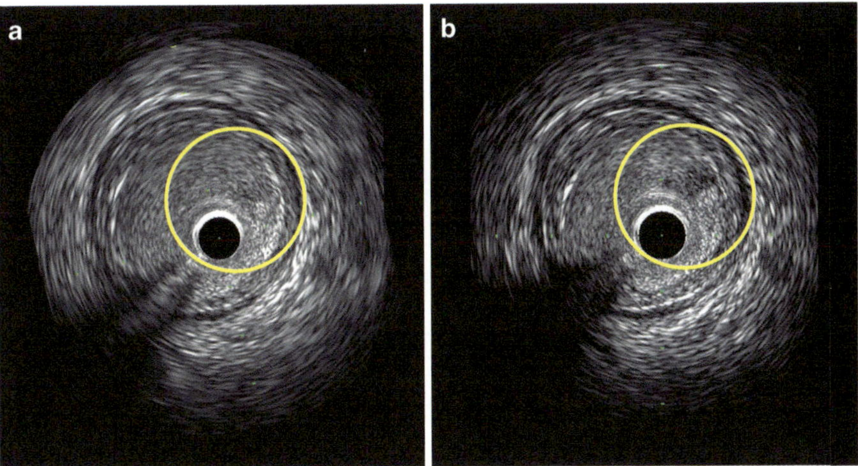

Fig. 7 Thrombus image in acute coronary syndrome. Thrombus was slightly more clearly delineated with 60 MHz IVUS (**b**) than with 40 MHz IVUS (**a**) (yellow circles)

4 Finally

The characteristics of thrombi on IVUS and the usefulness of IVUS in thrombotic lesions were discussed in this chapter. However, it is often difficult to distinguish between thrombus and plaque on IVUS, making quantitative evaluation difficult. In addition, we have not yet established a method for dealing with thrombus confirmed by IVUS. However, if advantages and disadvantages of IVUS can be well understood and its usefulness can be maximized, it will be useful for improving PCI outcomes.

References

1. Mintz GS, Nissen SE, Anderson WD, et al. American College of Cardiology Clinical Expert Consensus Document on standards for acquisition, measurement and reporting of intravascular ultrasound studies (IVUS). A report of the American College of Cardiology Task Force on clinical expert consensus documents. J Am Coll Cardiol. 2001;37:1478–92.
2. Hibi K, Kozuma K, Sonoda S, et al. A randomized study of distal filter protection versus conventional treatment during percutaneous coronary intervention in patients with attenuated plaque identified by intravascular ultrasound. JACC Cardiovasc Interv. 2018;11:1545–55.
3. Kramer MC, Verouden NC, Li X, et al. Thrombus aspiration alone during primary percutaneous coronary intervention as definitive treatment in acute ST-elevation myocardial infarction. Elevation myocardial infarction. Catheter Cardiovasc Interv. 2012;79:860–7.
4. Waldo SW, Armstrong EJ, Yeo KK, et al. Procedural success and long-term outcomes of aspiration thrombectomy for the treatment of stent thrombosis. Catheter Cardiovasc Interv. 2013;82:1048–53.

How to Evaluate Distal Vessel of the Culprit Lesion?

Hiroyuki Okura

Points for Comprehensive Utilization

- Causes of new stenoses at distal segments to the stent are coronary spasm, hematoma, and plaque shift.
- In lesions with persistent coronary spasm or shrinkage, the internal elastic membrane is wrinkled and recognized as PHB (perimedial high-echoic band) by IVUS.
- In patients with residual distal stenosis after treatment of CTO lesions, presence or absence of PHB can predict vessel enlargement in the chronic phase.

After stenting of the culprit lesion, IVUS should be evaluated not only for in-stent situation. IVUS is also useful in the evaluation of distal stent segments.

1 Assess the Distal Vessel Immediately after Stenting

Let us say that a new stenosis appeared in the distal part of the stent immediately after stent implantation. What would you think and how would you deal with it? Would you add a stent at that point if vasodilators did not change the situation? No, no, no. Wait a minute. Do we really need that stent?

H. Okura (✉)
Department of Cardiovascular Medicine, Gifu University Graduate School of Medicine, Gifu, Japan
e-mail: hokura@fides.dti.ne.jp

J. Honye (ed.), *Basics of Comprehensive IVUS-Guided PCI*,
https://doi.org/10.1007/978-981-19-5658-4_16

Here's the Trick

When a new stenosis appears after stenting, there are three probable causes.

1. Coronary spasm.
2. Stent edge dissection (~hematoma).
3. Stenosis caused by plaque shift.

If coronary spasm is persistent, it may not relieve with one or twice administration of vasodilators. If there is no chest pain, hypoperfusion, or ST-T changes, it is advisable to record IVUS once before immediate stenting. The same is true for residual stenosis in the distal vessel after dilatation of the culprit lesion for acute myocardial infarction.

Fig. 1 shows a case of acute myocardial infarction in which diffuse stenosis was observed in the distal vessel after stent implantation for the culprit lesion in the left main trunk. On coronary angiography immediately after stent implantation (Fig. 1a), there appeared to be residual stenosis in the distal left anterior descending artery. Since the stenosis did not improve despite intracoronary administration of isosorbide dinitrate, IVUS was performed (Fig. 1b). IVUS was performed (Fig. 1b). The diameter of the vessel was reduced considerably, and a

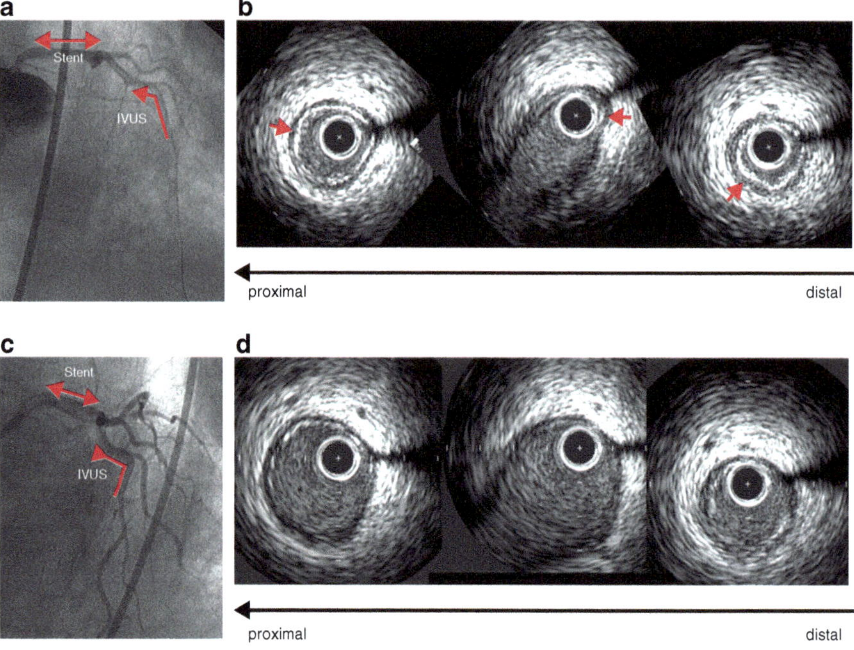

Fig. 1 A case of residual stenosis in the distal vessel immediately after stent implantation. (**a**) Coronary angiography immediately after stent implantation to the left main trunk. (**b**) IVUS image of the distal left anterior descending artery. (**c**) Coronary angiography after intracoronary nitroglycerin. (**d**) IVUS image at the same site as **b** after intracoronary nitroglycerin

high echoic band was observed in the luminal side of the low echogenic media (Fig. 1b arrow). Furthermore, selective intracoronary nitroglycerin administration relieved the stenosis (Fig. 1c), and repeat IVUS revealed markedly enlarged vessel diameter and decreased high echoic band. Histopathological examination revealed that media of the coronary artery wall thickens during coronary artery spasm, and the internal elastic membrane on the luminal side of media wrinkles (Fig. 2).

Fig. 3 shows a case in which stenosis appeared distally after stenting (Fig. 3a–c). Intracoronary administration of isosorbide nitrate did not improve the stenosis.

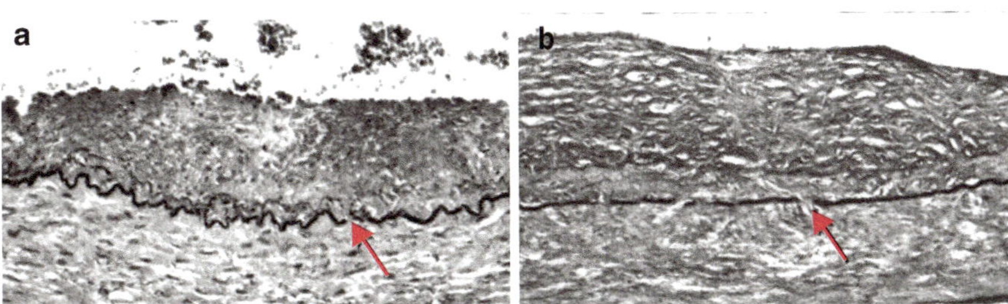

Fig. 2 Coronary spasm. (**a**) In coronary arteries during coronary spasm, the internal elastic membrane (arrow) is wrinkled. (**b**) In coronary arteries without coronary spasm, the internal elastic membrane (arrow) is not wrinkled

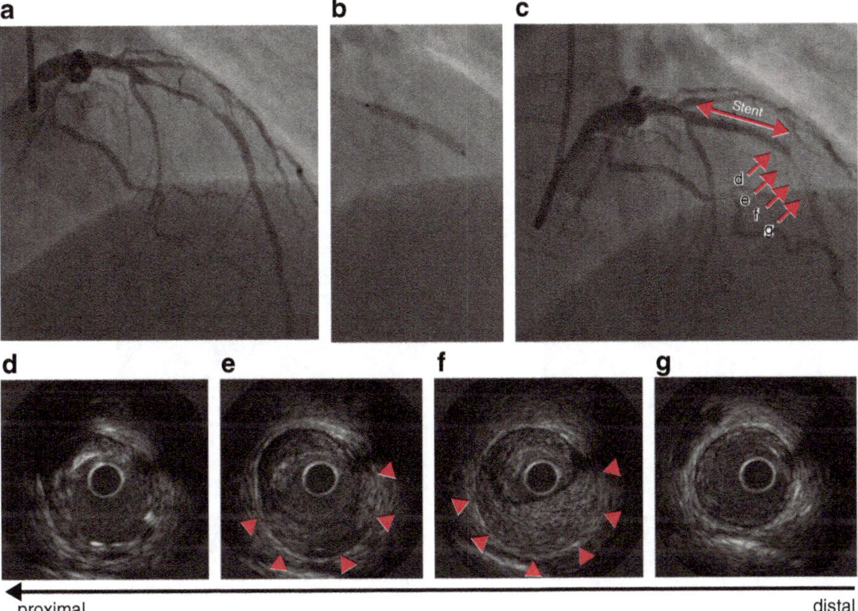

Fig. 3 Stent edge dissection. (**a**) Coronary angiography before stenting shows a tight stenosis in the left anterior descending artery. (**b**) Stent implantation. (**c**) Coronary angiography after stent implantation shows good dilatation at the stent site (arrow) but new stenosis appeared distally (arrow). IVUS pullback (**d**–**g**) from distal to the stent reveals a large intramural hematoma (arrowhead)

IVUS demonstrated a dissection at the stent edge and intramural hematoma distal to the dissection (Fig. 3d–g). In this case, an additional stent was placed and the stenosis improved.

2 Stenotic Lesions that Change during a Cardiac Cycle

Interesting findings on IVUS may also be seen in "distal segments" unrelated to stent implantation. In a left anterior descending artery, stenosis may not be present during diastole (arrow in Fig. 4a), but present only during systole (arrow in Fig. 4b). This is a myocardial bridge. When this area is observed by IVUS, the coronary artery is surrounded by a hypoechoic myocardial layer (Fig. 4c, d*), indicating that the coronary artery is compressed during systole. In addition, a high-echoic band on the luminal side of the media, which was not observed during diastole, can be clearly observed during systole (Fig. 4d arrowhead).

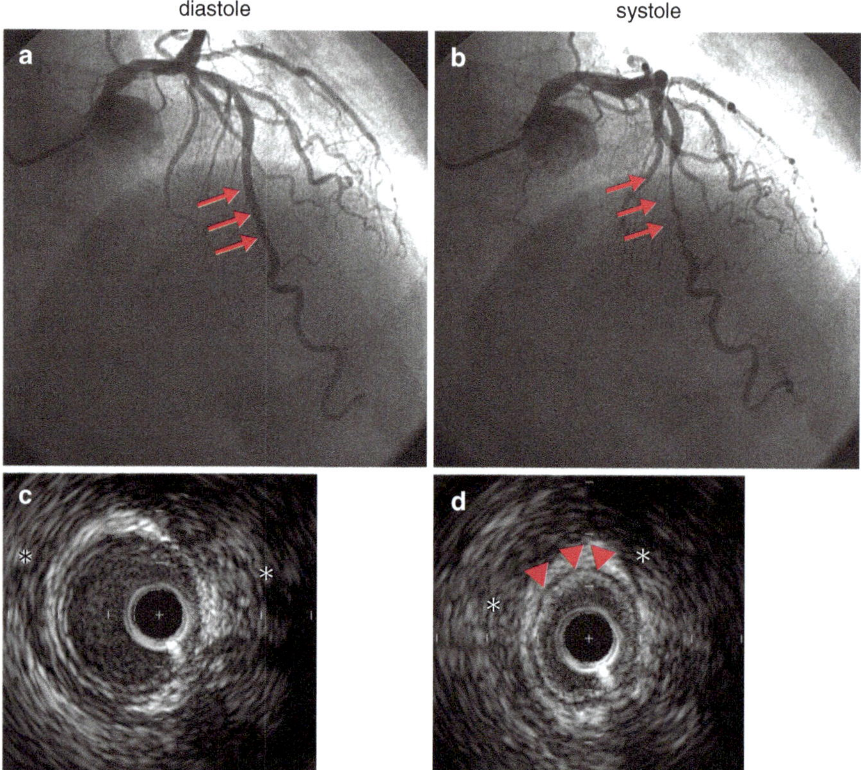

Fig. 4 Example of myocardial bridge. (**a**) No stenosis in the mid-left anterior descending artery (arrow) in diastole. (**b**) Severe stenosis in the same region in systole (arrow). (**c**) Hypoechoic myocardial tissue(*) surrounding the coronary artery on IVUS. (**d**) The coronary artery is compressed by myocardium in systole, and a high-echoic band (arrowhead) is seen on the luminal side of the media

3 Assess More Distal Vessels Immediately after Stenting

The greater the degree of stenosis of the culprit lesion, the lower the perfusion pressure in its distal segments and, consequently, the smaller the vessel size. A typical example of this finding is chronic total occlusion. The distal vessel of a CTO lesion will enlarge during the chronic phase in approximately 60–70% of lesions without additional treatment.

As mentioned above, it is known that the tunica media thickens and the inner elastic membrane wrinkles during coronary spasm [1, 2]. We thought that the high-intensity band observed on the luminal side of the tunica media on IVUS corresponds to the "wrinkles" of the internal elastic membrane, and named it peri-medial high echoic band (PHB) (Fig. 5 arrow) [3]. This finding is often seen in the culprit lesion of a CTO lesion or its distal vessel.

We compared changes in vessel diameter during the chronic phase in 26 tight stenotic lesions, including CTOs, between those with (PHB group) and without PHB (non-PHB group) in the distal vessel after stenting to the culprit lesion. In the PHB group, the vessel diameter was significantly enlarged, while in the group without PHB, the vessel diameter remained unchanged (Fig. 6). The presence of PHB on IVUS was the only independent predictor of vessel enlargement.

Fig. 7 shows a typical case. Three stents [XIENCE Alpine® (Abbott) 3.5 × 28 mm, 3.0 × 38 mm, and 2.5 × 38 mm, starting from the proximal part] were placed in the CTO lesion in the right coronary artery (Fig. 7a), and a diffuse stenosis remained in the distal vessel (Fig. 7b). IVUS showed circumferential PHB. No additional treatment was performed. One year later, vessel size increased and the stenosis disappeared (Fig. 7c).

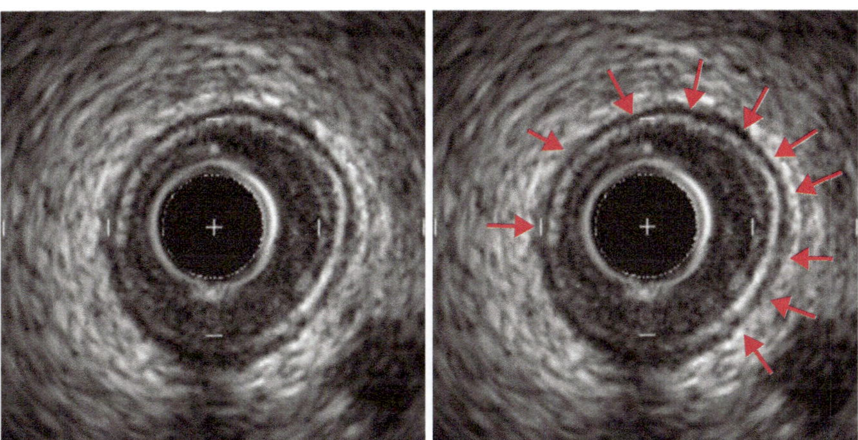

Fig. 5 Peri-medial high-echoic band (PHB). High echoic band (arrow) is seen on the luminal side of the hypoechoic tunica media in the coronary artery wall. This is referred to as PHB

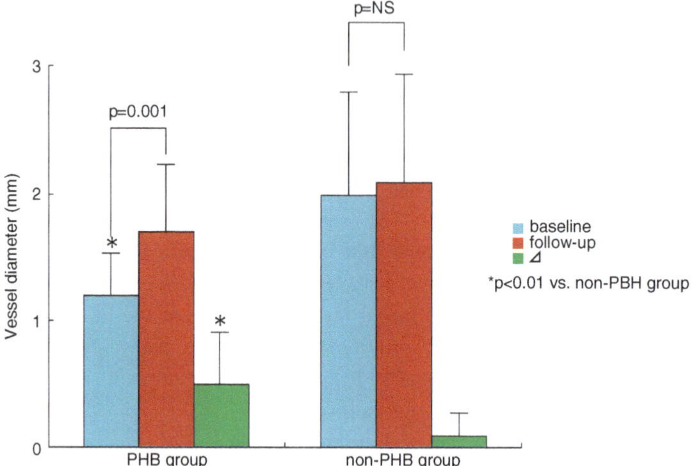

Fig. 6 Changes in vessel diameter over time in the distal part of the stent with PHB. In the PHB group, vessel diameter increased significantly in the chronic phase (follow-up) compared with immediate post-stenting phase (baseline), whereas no increase was observed in the non-PHB group. Vessel diameter (mm)

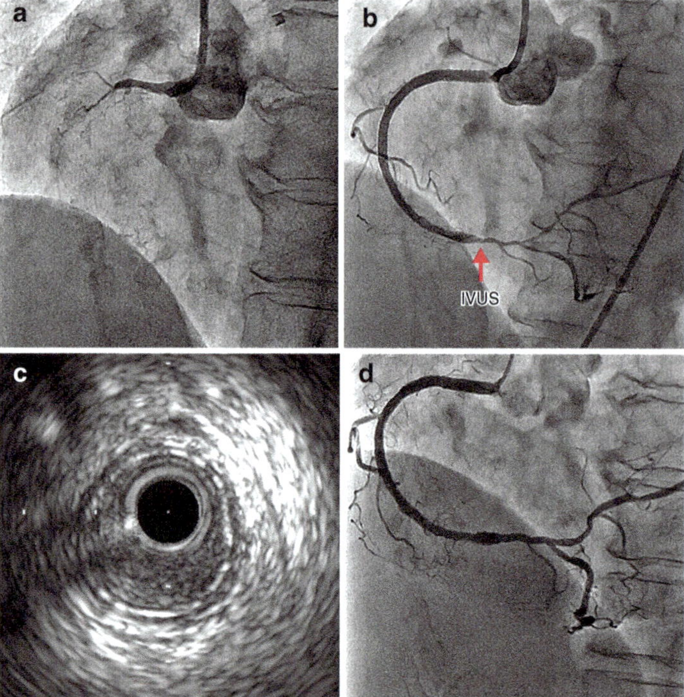

Fig. 7 A case of residual stenosis with PHB in the periphery after stenting of a CTO lesion in RCA (courtesy of Toyohashi Heart Center). (**a**) Pre-treatment. (**b**) Post-PCI. (**c**) 1-year follow-up. (**d**) IVUS images immediately after PCI. pre-treatment; After PCI; 1-year follow-up; IVUS

3.1 CTO: Chronic Total Occlusion

Advice

During PCI, operators tend to focus only on the stented area on IVUS, but further observation of the distal vessel may provide important information. The IVUS pullback should be performed at least 10 mm distally from the stent edge.

References

1. Mortensen ES, Rognum TO, Straume B, et al. Evidence at autopsy of spasm in the distal right coronary artery in persons with coronary heart disease dying suddenly. Cardiovasc Pathol. 2007;16:336–43.
2. Uchida Y, Matsuyama A, Koga A, et al. Functional medial thickening and folding of the internal elastic lamina in coronary spasm. Am J Physiol Heart Circ Physiol. 2011;300:H423–30.
3. Neishi Y, Okura H, Kume T, et al. Prediction of chronic vessel enlargement by a novel intravascular ultrasound finding. Circ J. 2015;79:607–12.

GPSR Compliance

The European Union's (EU) General Product Safety Regulation (GPSR) is a set of rules that requires consumer products to be safe and our obligations to ensure this.

If you have any concerns about our products, you can contact us on ProductSafety@springernature.com

In case Publisher is established outside the EU, the EU authorized representative is:

Springer Nature Customer Service Center GmbH
Europaplatz 3
69115 Heidelberg, Germany

Batch number: 10370708

Printed by Printforce, the Netherlands